Cram101 Textbook Outlines to accompany:

Essential Psychopharmacology

Stephen M. Stahl, 3rd Edition

A Content Technologies Inc. publication (c) 2012.

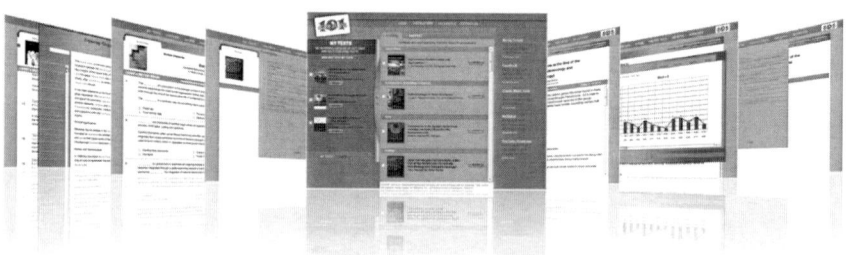

Learning System

Cram101 Textbook Outlines is a learning system. The notes in this book are the highlights of your textbook, you will never have to highlight a book again.

How to use this book. Take this book to class, it is your notebook for the lecture. The notes and highlights on the left hand side of the pages follow the outline and order of the textbook. All you have to do is follow along while your instructor presents the lecture. Circle the items emphasized in class and add other important information on the right side. With Cram101 Textbook Outlines you'll spend less time writing and more time listening. Learning becomes more efficient.

Cram101.com Online

Increase your studying efficiency by using Cram101.com's practice tests and online reference material. It is the perfect complement to Cram101 Textbook Outlines. Use self-teaching matching tests or simulate in-class testing with comprehensive multiple choice tests, or simply use Cram's true and false tests for quick review. Cram101.com even allows you to enter your in-class notes for an integrated studying format combining the textbook notes with your class notes.

Visit **www.Cram101.com**, click Sign Up at the top of the screen, and enter **DK73DW9525** in the promo code box on the registration screen. Your access to www.Cram101.com is discounted by 50% because you have purchased this book. Sign up and stop highlighting textbooks forever.

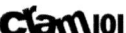

Essential Psychopharmacology
Stephen M. Stahl, 3rd

CONTENTS

Chapter 1. Structure and Function of Neurons

Symptom	A Symptom is a departure from normal function or feeling which is noticed by a patient, indicating the presence of disease or abnormality. A Symptom is subjective, observed by the patient, and not measured.
Atrophy	Atrophy is the partial or complete wasting away of a part of the body. Causes of Atrophy include poor nourishment, poor circulation, loss of hormonal support, loss of nerve supply to the target organ, disuse or lack of exercise or disease intrinsic to the tissue itself. Hormonal and nerve inputs that maintain an organ or body part are referred to as trophic [noun] in medical practice.
Axon	An axon is a long, slender projection of a nerve cell, or neuron, that conducts electrical impulses away from the neuron's cell body or soma. An axon is one of two types of protoplasmic protrusions that extrude from the cell body of a neuron, the other type being dendrites. Axons are distinguished from dendrites by several features, including shape (dendrites often taper while axons usually maintain a constant radius), length (dendrites are restricted to a small region around the cell body while axons can be much longer), and function (dendrites usually receive signals while axons usually transmit them).
Cannabinoid	Cannabinoids are a group of terpenophenolic compounds present in Cannabis (Cannabis sativa L) and which occur naturally in the nervous and immune systems of animals. The broader definition of Cannabinoids refers to a group of substances that are structurally related to tetrahydrocannabinol (THC) or that bind to Cannabinoid receptors. The chemical definition encompasses a variety of distinct chemical classes: the classical Cannabinoids structurally related to THC, the nonclassical Cannabinoids, the aminoalkylindoles, the eicosanoids related to the endoCannabinoids, 1,5-diarylpyrazoles, quinolines and arylsulphonamides and additional compounds that do not fall into these standard classes but bind to Cannabinoid receptors.
Glucocorticoid	Glucocorticoids (GC) are a class of steroid hormones that bind to the Glucocorticoid receptor (GR), which is present in almost every vertebrate animal cell. The name Glucocorticoid derives from their role in the regulation of the metabolism of glucose, their synthesis in the adrenal cortex, and their steroidal structure . GCs are part of the feedback mechanism in the immune system that turns immune activity (inflammation) down.

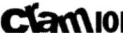

Chapter 1. Structure and Function of Neurons

Histamine	Histamine is a biogenic amine involved in local immune responses as well as regulating physiological function in the gut and acting as a neurotransmitter. Histamine triggers the inflammatory response. As part of an immune response to foreign pathogens, Histamine is produced by basophils and by mast cells found in nearby connective tissues.
Hypnotic	Benzodiazepines are the most well known and most frequently prescribed Hypnotic medication presently. However, their use in recent years is being increasingly replaced by newer nonbenzodiazepine Hypnotic drugs and the hormone melatonin, which in North America is called a 'supplement'. Benzodiazepines are effective in the short term but with long term use beyond 1 - 2 weeks tolerance to their Hypnotic effects develops thus making them ineffective for long term use.
Presenilin	Presenilins are a family of related multi-pass transmembrane proteins that function as a part of the gamma-secretase protease complex. Vertebrates have two Presenilin genes, called PSEN1 (located on chromosome 14 in humans) that encodes Presenilin 1 (PS-1) and PSEN2 (on chromosome 1 in humans) that codes for Presenilin 2 (PS-2). Both genes show conservation between species, with little difference between rat and human Presenilins.
Receptor	In biochemistry, a receptor is a protein molecule, embedded in either the plasma membrane or the cytoplasm of a cell, to which one or more specific kinds of signaling molecules may attach. A molecule which binds (attaches) to a receptor is called a ligand, and may be a peptide (short protein) or other small molecule, such as a neurotransmitter, a hormone, a pharmaceutical drug, or a toxin. Each kind of receptor can bind only certain ligand shapes.
Soma	Soma from Proto-Indo-Iranian *sauma-, was a ritual drink of importance among the early Indo-Iranians, and the later Vedic and greater Persian cultures. It is frequently mentioned in the Rigveda, whose Soma Mandala contains many hymns praising its energizing qualities. In the Avesta, Haoma has an entire Yasht dedicated to it.
Syndrome	In medicine and psychology, a Syndrome is the association of several clinically recognizable features, signs (observed by a physician), symptoms (reported by the patient), phenomena or characteristics that often occur together, so that the presence of one feature alerts the physician to the presence of the others. In recent decades, the term has been used outside medicine to refer to a combination of phenomena seen in association. The term Syndrome derives from its Greek roots and means literally 'run together', as the features do.

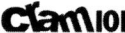

Chapter 1. Structure and Function of Neurons

Adrenergic receptors	The Adrenergic receptors are a class of G protein-coupled receptors that are targets of the catecholamines, especially noradrenaline (norepinephrine) and adrenaline (epinephrine). Although dopamine is a catecholamine, its receptors are in a different category. Many cells possess these receptors, and the binding of an agonist will generally cause a sympathetic response (e.g. the fight-or-flight response). For instance, the heart rate will increase and the pupils will dilate, energy will be mobilized, and blood flow diverted from other non-essential organs to skeletal muscle.
Agonist	An Agonist is a drug that binds to a receptor of a cell and triggers a response by the cell. An Agonist often mimics the action of a naturally occurring substance. An Agonist produces an action.
Amino acid	Amino acids are molecules containing an amine group, a carboxylic acid group and a side-chain that varies between different amino acids. The key elements of an amino acid are carbon, hydrogen, oxygen, and nitrogen. They are particularly important in biochemistry, where the term usually refers to alpha-amino acids.
Antipsychotic	An antipsychotic is a tranquilizing psychiatric medication primarily used to manage psychosis (including delusions or hallucinations, as well as disordered thought), particularly in schizophrenia and bipolar disorder. A first generation of antipsychotics, known as typical antipsychotics, was discovered in the 1950s. Most of the drugs in the second generation, known as atypical antipsychotics, have been developed more recently, although the first atypical antipsychotic, clozapine, was discovered in the 1950s and introduced clinically in the 1970s.
Atypical antipsychotics	The Atypical antipsychotics are a group of antipsychotic drugs used to treat psychiatric conditions. Some Atypical antipsychotics are FDA approved for use in the treatment of schizophrenia. Some carry FDA approved indications for acute mania, bipolar mania, psychotic agitation, bipolar maintenance, and other indications.
Calcium	Calcium is the chemical element with the symbol Ca and atomic number 20. It has an atomic mass of 40.078 amu. Calcium is a soft gray alkaline earth metal, and is the fifth most abundant element by mass in the Earth's crust. Calcium is also the fifth most abundant dissolved ion in seawater by both molarity and mass, after sodium, chloride, magnesium, and sulfate.

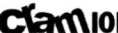

Chapter 1. Structure and Function of Neurons

Huntington's disease	Huntington's disease is a neurodegenerative genetic disorder that affects muscle coordination and leads to cognitive decline and dementia. It typically becomes noticeable in middle age. Huntington's disease is the most common genetic cause of abnormal involuntary writhing movements called chorea.
Norepinephrine	Noradrenaline (BAN) is a catecholamine with dual roles as a hormone and a neurotransmitter. As a stress hormone, Norepinephrine affects parts of the brain where attention and responding actions are controlled. Along with epinephrine, Norepinephrine also underlies the fight-or-flight response, directly increasing heart rate, triggering the release of glucose from energy stores, and increasing blood flow to skeletal muscle.
Oxidoreductase	In biochemistry, an Oxidoreductase is an enzyme that catalyzes the transfer of electrons from one molecule (the reductant, also called the hydrogen or electron donor) to another (the oxidant, also called the hydrogen or electron acceptor).
Schizophrenia	Schizophrenia , from the Greek roots skhizein and phrÄ"n, phren- (φρÎ®ν, φρεν-; 'mind') is a psychiatric diagnosis that describes a neuropsychiatric and mental disorder characterized by abnormalities in the perception or expression of reality. It most commonly manifests as auditory hallucinations, paranoid or bizarre delusions, or disorganized speech and thinking with significant social or occupational dysfunction. Onset of symptoms typically occurs in young adulthood, with around 0.4-0.6% of the population affected.
Serotonin	Serotonin is a monoamine neurotransmitter. Biochemically derived from tryptophan, serotonin is primarily found in the gastrointestinal (GI) tract, platelets, and in the central nervous system (CNS) of animals including humans. It is a well-known contributor to feelings of well-being; therefore it is also known as a 'happiness hormone' despite not being a hormone.
Benadryl	Benadryl is a brand name allergy medicine marketed over-the-counter by Johnson ' Johnson subsidiary McNeil Consumer Healthcare. Prior to 2007, Benadryl was marketed by Pfizer Consumer Healthcare. Benadryl is used as an antihistamine for the temporary relief of seasonal and perennial allergy symptoms.
Amyloid	Amyloids are insoluble fibrous protein aggregates sharing specific structural traits. Abnormal accumulation of amyloid in organs may lead to amyloidosis, and may play a role in various neurodegenerative diseases.

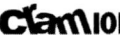

Chapter 1. Structure and Function of Neurons

	The name amyloid comes from the early mistaken identification of the substance as starch, based on crude iodine-staining techniques.
Cerebellum	The Cerebellum is a region of the brain that plays an important role in motor control. It is also involved in some cognitive functions such as attention and language, and probably in some emotional functions such as regulating fear and pleasure responses, but its function in movement is the most clearly understood. The Cerebellum does not initiate movement, but it contributes to coordination, precision, and accurate timing.
Excitotoxicity	Excitotoxicity is the pathological process by which nerve cells are damaged and killed by glutamate and similar substances. This occurs when receptors for the excitatory neurotransmitter glutamate (glutamate receptors) such as the NMDA receptor and AMPA receptor are overactivated. Excitotoxins like NMDA and kainic acid which bind to these receptors, as well as pathologically high levels of glutamate, can cause Excitotoxicity by allowing high levels of calcium ions (Ca^{2+}) to enter the cell.
Sedation	Sedation is a medical procedure involving the administration of sedative drugs, generally to facilitate a medical procedure or diagnostic proceedure. Drugs which can be used for Sedation include propofol, etomidate, ketamine, fentanyl and midazolam.
Aventyl	Nortriptyline is a second-generation tricyclic antidepressant marketed as the hydrochloride under the trade names Sensoval, Aventyl, Pamelor, Norpress, Allegron and Nortrilen. It is used in the treatment of major depression and childhood nocturnal enuresis (bedwetting). In addition, it is sometimes used for chronic illnesses such as chronic fatigue syndrome, chronic pain and migraines, and labile affect in some neurological conditions.
Cerebrospinal fluid	Cerebrospinal fluid Liquor cerebrospinalis, is a clear bodily fluid that occupies the subarachnoid space and the ventricular system around and inside the brain. In essence, the brain 'floats' in it. The CSF occupies the space between the arachnoid mater (the middle layer of the brain cover, meninges), and the pia mater (the layer of the meninges closest to the brain).
Somatic	The term somatic means 'of the body'. It is often used in biology to refer to the cells of the body in contrast to the cells in the germline which give rise to the gametes (eggs or sperm). These somatic cells are diploid containing two copies of each chromosome, whereas the germ cells are haploid as they only contain one copy of each chromosome.

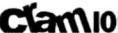

Chapter 1. Structure and Function of Neurons

Tyramine	Tyramine is a naturally-occurring monoamine compound and trace amine derived from the amino acid tyrosine. Tyramine acts as a catecholamine (dopamine, norepinephrine (noradrenaline), epinephrine (adrenaline)) releasing agent. Notably, however, it is unable to cross the blood-brain-barrier (BBB), resulting in only non-psychoactive peripheral sympathomimetic effects.
Amitriptyline	Amitriptyline is a psychoactive drug and pharmaceutical of the tricyclic antidepressant (TCA) chemical class which is used primarily as an antidepressant and anxiolytic agent. It is the most widely prescribed TCA and perhaps also the most efficient against depressive symptoms. Amitriptyline is approved for the treatment of major depression.
Prolixin	Fluphenazine is a typical antipsychotic drug used for the treatment of psychoses such as schizophrenia and acute manic phases of bipolar disorder. It belongs to the piperazine class of phenothiazines and is extremely potent; more potent than haloperidol and around fifty to seventy times the potency of chlorpromazine. It is marketed under the brand name of Prolixin and Sydocate(Surge Laboratories).
Dopamine	Dopamine is a neurotransmitter that occurs in a wide variety of animals, including both vertebrates and invertebrates. In the brain, this phenethylamine functions as a neurotransmitter, activating the five types of Dopamine receptors--D_1, D_2, D_3, D_4, and D_5--and their variants. Dopamine is produced in several areas of the brain, including the substantia nigra and the ventral tegmental area.
Interaction	Interaction is a kind of action that occurs as two or more objects have an effect upon one another. The idea of a two-way effect is essential in the concept of Interaction, as opposed to a one-way causal effect. A closely related term is interconnectivity, which deals with the Interactions of Interactions within systems: combinations of many simple Interactions can lead to surprising emergent phenomena.
Peptide	Peptides are short polymers formed from the linking, in a defined order, of α-amino acids. The link between one amino acid residue and the next is called an amide bond or a Peptide bond. Proteins are polyPeptide molecules, or consist of multiple polyPeptide subunits, each composed of chains containing a specific sequence of the 22 proteinogenic amino acids.

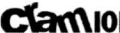

Chapter 1. Structure and Function of Neurons

Peptide synthesis	In organic chemistry, Peptide synthesis is the production of peptides, which are organic compounds in which multiple amino acids are linked via peptide bonds which are also known as amide bonds. The biological process of producing long peptides (proteins) is known as protein biosynthesis. Peptides are synthesized by coupling the carboxyl group or C-terminus of one amino acid to the amino group or N-terminus of another.
Psychopharmacology	Psychopharmacology is the study of drug-induced changes in mood, sensation, thinking, and behavior. The field of Psychopharmacology studies a wide range of substances with various types of psychoactive properties. The professional and commercial fields of pharmacology and Psychopharmacology do not mainly focus on psychedelic or recreational drugs, as the majority of studies are conducted for the development, study, and use of drugs for the modification of behavior and the alleviation of symptoms, particularly in the treatment of mental disorders .
Abuse	Abuse is defined as:
Antidepressant	An antidepressant is a psychiatric medication used to alleviate mood disorders, such as major depression and dysthymia and anxiety disorders such as social anxiety disorder. According to Gelder, Mayou '*Geddes (2005) people with a depressive illness will experience a therapeutic effect to their mood, however this will not be experienced in healthy individuals. Drugs including the monoamine oxidase inhibitors (MAOIs), tricyclic antidepressants (TCAs), tetracyclic antidepressants (TeCAs), selective serotonin reuptake inhibitors (SSRIs), and serotonin-norepinephrine reuptake inhibitors (SNRIs) are most commonly associated with the term.
Cocaine	Cocaine is a crystalline tropane alkaloid that is obtained from the leaves of the coca plant. The name comes from 'coca' in addition to the alkaloid suffix -ine, forming Cocaine. It is a stimulant of the central nervous system and an appetite suppressant.
Stimulants	Stimulants, also sometimes called psychoStimulants, are psychoactive drugs which induce temporary improvements in either mental or physical function or both. Examples of these kinds of effects may include enhanced alertness, wakefulness, and locomotion, among others. Due to their effects typically having an 'up' quality to them, Stimulants are also occasionally referred to as 'uppers'.

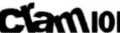

Chapter 2. Synaptic Neurotransmission and the Nervous System

Symptom	A Symptom is a departure from normal function or feeling which is noticed by a patient, indicating the presence of disease or abnormality. A Symptom is subjective, observed by the patient, and not measured.
Nervous system	The Nervous system is an organ system containing a network of specialized cells called neurons that coordinate the actions of an animal and transmit signals between different parts of its body. In most animals the Nervous system consists of two parts, central and peripheral. The central Nervous system contains the brain and spinal cord.
Huntington's disease	Huntington's disease is a neurodegenerative genetic disorder that affects muscle coordination and leads to cognitive decline and dementia. It typically becomes noticeable in middle age. Huntington's disease is the most common genetic cause of abnormal involuntary writhing movements called chorea.
Psychopharmacology	Psychopharmacology is the study of drug-induced changes in mood, sensation, thinking, and behavior.
	The field of Psychopharmacology studies a wide range of substances with various types of psychoactive properties. The professional and commercial fields of pharmacology and Psychopharmacology do not mainly focus on psychedelic or recreational drugs, as the majority of studies are conducted for the development, study, and use of drugs for the modification of behavior and the alleviation of symptoms, particularly in the treatment of mental disorders .
Probability	Probability is a way of expressing knowledge or belief that an event will occur or has occurred. The concept has an exact mathematical meaning in probability theory, which is used extensively in such areas of study as mathematics, statistics, finance, gambling, science, artificial intelligence/machine learning and philosophy to draw conclusions about the likelihood of potential events and the underlying mechanics of complex systems.
Stem cell	Stem cells are cells found in most, if not all, multi-cellular organisms. They are characterized by the ability to renew themselves through mitotic cell division and differentiating into a diverse range of specialized cell types. Research in the Stem cell field grew out of findings by Canadian scientists Ernest A. McCulloch and James E. Till in the 1960s.
Estrogen	Estrogens (U.S., otherwise oEstrogens or Å"strogens) are a group of steroid compounds and functioning as the primary female sex hormone, their name comes from estrus/oistros (period of fertility for female mammals) + gen/gonos = to generate.

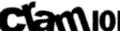

Chapter 2. Synaptic Neurotransmission and the Nervous System

	Estrogens are used as part of some oral contraceptives, in Estrogen replacement therapy for postmenopausal women, and in hormone replacement therapy for trans women.
	Like all steroid hormones, Estrogens readily diffuse across the cell membrane.
Necrosis	Necrosis is the premature death of cells and living tissue. Necrosis is caused by external factors, such as infection, toxins or trauma. This is in contrast to apoptosis, which is a naturally occurring cause of cellular death.
Syndrome	In medicine and psychology, a Syndrome is the association of several clinically recognizable features, signs (observed by a physician), symptoms (reported by the patient), phenomena or characteristics that often occur together, so that the presence of one feature alerts the physician to the presence of the others. In recent decades, the term has been used outside medicine to refer to a combination of phenomena seen in association.
	The term Syndrome derives from its Greek roots and means literally 'run together', as the features do.
Atrophy	Atrophy is the partial or complete wasting away of a part of the body. Causes of Atrophy include poor nourishment, poor circulation, loss of hormonal support, loss of nerve supply to the target organ, disuse or lack of exercise or disease intrinsic to the tissue itself. Hormonal and nerve inputs that maintain an organ or body part are referred to as trophic [noun] in medical practice.
Dopamine	Dopamine is a neurotransmitter that occurs in a wide variety of animals, including both vertebrates and invertebrates. In the brain, this phenethylamine functions as a neurotransmitter, activating the five types of Dopamine receptors--D_1, D_2, D_3, D_4, and D_5--and their variants. Dopamine is produced in several areas of the brain, including the substantia nigra and the ventral tegmental area.
Epilepsy	Epilepsy is a common chronic neurological disorder characterized by recurrent unprovoked seizures. These seizures are transient signs and/or symptoms of abnormal, excessive or synchronous neuronal activity in the brain. About 50 million people worldwide have Epilepsy, with almost 90% of these people being in developing countries.

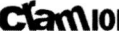

Chapter 2. Synaptic Neurotransmission and the Nervous System

Schizophrenia	Schizophrenia , from the Greek roots skhizein and phrÄ"n, phren- (φρÎ®ν, φρεν-; 'mind') is a psychiatric diagnosis that describes a neuropsychiatric and mental disorder characterized by abnormalities in the perception or expression of reality. It most commonly manifests as auditory hallucinations, paranoid or bizarre delusions, or disorganized speech and thinking with significant social or occupational dysfunction. Onset of symptoms typically occurs in young adulthood, with around 0.4-0.6% of the population affected.
Attention deficit hyperactivity disorder	Attention deficit hyperactivity disorder is a developmental disorder. It is primarily characterized by 'the co-existence of attentional problems and hyperactivity, with each behavior occurring infrequently alone' and symptoms starting before seven years of age.
	Attention deficit hyperactivity disorder is the most commonly studied and diagnosed psychiatric disorder in children, affecting about 3 to 5 percent of children globally and diagnosed in about 2 to 16 percent of school aged children.
Fibromyalgia	Fibromyalgia is also referred to as FM or FMS. Fibromyalgia is characterized by chronic widespread pain and allodynia, a heightened and painful response to pressure.
Hormone	A hormone is a chemical released by one or more cells that affects cells in other parts of the organism. Only a small amount of hormone is required to alter cell metabolism. It is essentially a chemical messenger that transports a signal from one cell to another.
Menstrual cycle	The menstrual cycle is the scientific term for the physiological changes that can occur in fertile female humans and apes. Overt menstruation (where there is blood flow from the uterus through the vagina) occurs in humans and some animals such as chimpanzees. Females of other species of placental mammal undergo estrous cycles, in which the endometrium is completely reabsorbed by the animal (covert menstruation) at the end of its reproductive cycle.
Neurotrophin	Neurotrophins are a family of proteins that induce the survival, development, and function of neurons.
	They belong to a class of growth factors, secreted proteins that are capable of signaling particular cells to survive, differentiate, or grow. Growth factors such as neurotrophins that promote the survival of neurons are known as neurotrophic factors.

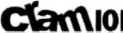

Chapter 2. Synaptic Neurotransmission and the Nervous System

Receptor	In biochemistry, a receptor is a protein molecule, embedded in either the plasma membrane or the cytoplasm of a cell, to which one or more specific kinds of signaling molecules may attach. A molecule which binds (attaches) to a receptor is called a ligand, and may be a peptide (short protein) or other small molecule, such as a neurotransmitter, a hormone, a pharmaceutical drug, or a toxin. Each kind of receptor can bind only certain ligand shapes.
Cytokine	Cytokines are small cell-signaling protein molecules that are secreted by the glial cells of the nervous system and by numerous cells of the immune system and are a category of signaling molecules used extensively in intercellular communication. Cytokines can be classified as proteins, peptides, or glycoproteins; the term 'cytokine' encompasses a large and diverse family of regulators produced throughout the body by cells of diverse embryological origin.
Radicals	In chemistry, radicals are atoms, molecules, or ions with unpaired electrons on an open shell configuration. The unpaired electrons cause them to be highly chemically reactive. radicals play an important role in combustion, atmospheric chemistry, polymerization, plasma chemistry, biochemistry, and many other chemical processes, including human physiology.
Abuse	Abuse is defined as:
Antibiotic	In common usage, an Antibiotic is a substance or compound that kills, or inhibits the growth of, bacteria. Antibiotics belong to the broader group of antimicrobial compounds, used to treat infections caused by microorganisms, including fungi and protozoa.

The term 'Antibiotic' was coined by Selman Waksman in 1942 to describe any substance produced by a microorganism that is antagonistic to the growth of other microorganisms in high dilution. |
| Atorvastatin | Atorvastatin is a member of the drug class known as statins, used for lowering blood cholesterol. It also stabilizes plaque and prevents strokes through anti-inflammatory and other mechanisms.

Atorvastatin inhibits HMG-CoA reductase, the rate-determining enzyme located in hepatic tissue that produces mevalonate, a small molecule used in the synthesis of cholesterol and other mevalonate derivatives. This lowers the amount of cholesterol produced which in turn lowers the total amount of LDL cholesterol. Atorvastatin was first synthesized in 1985 by Bruce Roth while working at Parke-Davis Warner-Lambert Company (now Pfizer). |

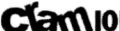

Chapter 2. Synaptic Neurotransmission and the Nervous System

Huntington's disease	Huntington's disease is a neurodegenerative genetic disorder that affects muscle coordination and leads to cognitive decline and dementia. It typically becomes noticeable in middle age. Huntington's disease is the most common genetic cause of abnormal involuntary writhing movements called chorea.
Erythromycin	Erythromycin is a macrolide antibiotic that has an antimicrobial spectrum similar to or slightly wider than that of penicillin, and is often used for people who have an allergy to penicillins. For respiratory tract infections, it has better coverage of atypical organisms, including mycoplasma and Legionellosis. It was first marketed by Eli Lilly and Company, and it is today commonly known as EES (Erythromycin ethylsuccinate, an ester prodrug that is commonly administered).
Macrolide	The macrolides are a group of drugs (typically antibiotics) whose activity stems from the presence of a macrolide ring, a large macrocyclic lactone ring to which one or more deoxy sugars, usually cladinose and desosamine, may be attached. The lactone rings are usually 14, 15 or 16-membered. macrolides belong to the polyketide class of natural products. · Azithromycin (Zithromax, Zitromax, Sumamed, Azitrox) - Unique, does not inhibit CYP3A4 · Clarithromycin (Biaxin, Fromilid, Klacid, Klabax, Lekoklar) · Dirithromycin (Dynabac) · Erythromycin · Roxithromycin (Rulid, Surlid,Roxid) · Telithromycin · Carbomycin A · Josamycin · Kitasamycin

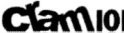

· Midecamicine/midecamicine acetate

· Oleandomycin

· Spiramycin

· Troleandomycin

· Tylosin/tylocine (Tylan)

Ketolides are a new class of antibiotics that are structurally related to the macrolides.

Mood stabilizer	A Mood stabilizer is a psychiatric medication used to treat mood disorders characterized by intense and sustained mood shifts, which is not the same as 'feeling good one minute and then bad the next.' One use is in bipolar disorder, where Mood stabilizers suppress swings between mania and depression. These drugs are also used in borderline personality disorder. Most Mood stabilizers are purely antimanic agents, meaning that they are effective at treating mania and mood cycling and shifting, but are not effective at treating depression.
Simvastatin	Simvastatin is a hypolipidemic drug belonging to the class of pharmaceuticals called 'statins'. It is used to control hypercholesterolemia (elevated cholesterol levels) and to prevent cardiovascular disease. Simvastatin is a synthetic derivate of a fermentation product of Aspergillus terreus.
Triazolam	Triazolam is a benzodiazepine derivative drug. It possesses pharmacological properties similar to that of other benzodiazepines, but it is generally only used as a sedative to treat insomnia. In addition to the hypnotic properties Triazolam possesses, amnesic, anxiolytic, sedative, anticonvulsant and muscle relaxant properties are also present.

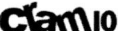

Chapter 2. Synaptic Neurotransmission and the Nervous System

Aventyl	Nortriptyline is a second-generation tricyclic antidepressant marketed as the hydrochloride under the trade names Sensoval, Aventyl, Pamelor, Norpress, Allegron and Nortrilen. It is used in the treatment of major depression and childhood nocturnal enuresis (bedwetting). In addition, it is sometimes used for chronic illnesses such as chronic fatigue syndrome, chronic pain and migraines, and labile affect in some neurological conditions.
Enzyme	Enzymes are proteins that catalyze (i.e., increase the rates of) chemical reactions. In enzymatic reactions, the molecules at the beginning of the process are called substrates, and the Enzyme converts them into different molecules, called the products. Almost all processes in a biological cell need Enzymes to occur at significant rates.
Neurotransmitters	Neurotransmitters are endogenous chemicals which relay, amplify, and modulate signals between a neuron and another cell. Neurotransmitters are packaged into synaptic vesicles that cluster beneath the membrane on the presynaptic side of a synapse, and are released into the synaptic cleft, where they bind to receptors in the membrane on the postsynaptic side of the synapse. Release of Neurotransmitters usually follows arrival of an action potential at the synapse, but may follow graded electrical potentials.
Excitotoxicity	Excitotoxicity is the pathological process by which nerve cells are damaged and killed by glutamate and similar substances. This occurs when receptors for the excitatory neurotransmitter glutamate (glutamate receptors) such as the NMDA receptor and AMPA receptor are overactivated. Excitotoxins like NMDA and kainic acid which bind to these receptors, as well as pathologically high levels of glutamate, can cause Excitotoxicity by allowing high levels of calcium ions (Ca^{2+}) to enter the cell.

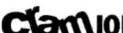

Chapter 3. Signal Transduction and the Chemically Addressed Nervous System

Symptom	A Symptom is a departure from normal function or feeling which is noticed by a patient, indicating the presence of disease or abnormality. A Symptom is subjective, observed by the patient, and not measured.
Agonist	An Agonist is a drug that binds to a receptor of a cell and triggers a response by the cell. An Agonist often mimics the action of a naturally occurring substance. An Agonist produces an action.
Mirtazapine	Mirtazapine is a psychoactive drug of the benzazepine and tetracyclic antidepressant (TeCA) chemical classes which is used primarily as an antidepressant. It is sometimes used for its anxiolytic, hypnotic, antiemetic, orexigenic, and antihistamine or antipruritic effects. Mirtazapine was introduced by Organon International in 1994. Along with its chemical analogue and predecessor mianserin (Bolvidon, Norval, Tolvon), Mirtazapine is one of the few noradrenergic and specific serotonergic antidepressants (NaSSAs).
Neurotransmitters	Neurotransmitters are endogenous chemicals which relay, amplify, and modulate signals between a neuron and another cell. Neurotransmitters are packaged into synaptic vesicles that cluster beneath the membrane on the presynaptic side of a synapse, and are released into the synaptic cleft, where they bind to receptors in the membrane on the postsynaptic side of the synapse. Release of Neurotransmitters usually follows arrival of an action potential at the synapse, but may follow graded electrical potentials.
Receptor	In biochemistry, a receptor is a protein molecule, embedded in either the plasma membrane or the cytoplasm of a cell, to which one or more specific kinds of signaling molecules may attach. A molecule which binds (attaches) to a receptor is called a ligand, and may be a peptide (short protein) or other small molecule, such as a neurotransmitter, a hormone, a pharmaceutical drug, or a toxin. Each kind of receptor can bind only certain ligand shapes.
Serotonin	Serotonin is a monoamine neurotransmitter. Biochemically derived from tryptophan, serotonin is primarily found in the gastrointestinal (GI) tract, platelets, and in the central nervous system (CNS) of animals including humans. It is a well-known contributor to feelings of well-being; therefore it is also known as a 'happiness hormone' despite not being a hormone.
Serotonin receptors	The serotonin receptors also known as 5-hydroxytryptamine receptors or 5-HT receptors are a group of G protein-coupled receptors (GPCRs) and ligand-gated ion channels (LGICs) found in the central and peripheral nervous systems. They mediate both excitatory and inhibitory neurotransmission. The serotonin receptors are activated by the neurotransmitter serotonin, which acts as their natural ligand.

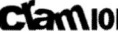

Chapter 3. Signal Transduction and the Chemically Addressed Nervous System

Benadryl	Benadryl is a brand name allergy medicine marketed over-the-counter by Johnson ' Johnson subsidiary McNeil Consumer Healthcare. Prior to 2007, Benadryl was marketed by Pfizer Consumer Healthcare. Benadryl is used as an antihistamine for the temporary relief of seasonal and perennial allergy symptoms.
Amitriptyline	Amitriptyline is a psychoactive drug and pharmaceutical of the tricyclic antidepressant (TCA) chemical class which is used primarily as an antidepressant and anxiolytic agent. It is the most widely prescribed TCA and perhaps also the most efficient against depressive symptoms. Amitriptyline is approved for the treatment of major depression.
Psychopharmacology	Psychopharmacology is the study of drug-induced changes in mood, sensation, thinking, and behavior. The field of Psychopharmacology studies a wide range of substances with various types of psychoactive properties. The professional and commercial fields of pharmacology and Psychopharmacology do not mainly focus on psychedelic or recreational drugs, as the majority of studies are conducted for the development, study, and use of drugs for the modification of behavior and the alleviation of symptoms, particularly in the treatment of mental disorders .
Valium	Diazepam , first marketed as Valium by Hoffmann-La Roche, is a benzodiazepine derivative drug. It is commonly used for treating anxiety, insomnia, seizures, muscle spasms, restless legs syndrome, alcohol withdrawal, benzodiazepine withdrawal, and Ménière's disease. It may also be used before certain medical procedures to reduce tension and anxiety, and in some surgical procedures to induce amnesia.
Alprazolam	Alprazolam, also known under the trade names Xanax (not to be confused with Zantac), Xanor, Alprax, and Niravam, is a short-acting drug of the benzodiazepine class. It is primarily used to treat moderate to severe anxiety disorders and panic attacks, and is used as an adjunctive treatment for anxiety associated with moderate depression. It is also available in an extended-release form, Xanax XR, both of which are now available in generic form. Alprazolam possesses anxiolytic, sedative, hypnotic, anticonvulsant, and muscle relaxant properties.
Calcium	Calcium is the chemical element with the symbol Ca and atomic number 20. It has an atomic mass of 40.078 amu. Calcium is a soft gray alkaline earth metal, and is the fifth most abundant element by mass in the Earth's crust. Calcium is also the fifth most abundant dissolved ion in seawater by both molarity and mass, after sodium, chloride, magnesium, and sulfate.

Chapter 3. Signal Transduction and the Chemically Addressed Nervous System

Calcium channel	A Calcium channel is an ion channel which displays selective permeabiltiy to calcium ions. It is sometimes synonymous as voltage-dependent Calcium channel, although there are also ligand-gated Calcium channels. The following tables explain gating, gene, location and function of different types of Calcium channels, both voltage and ligand-gated. · the receptor-operated Calcium channels (in vasoconstriction) · P2X receptor Calcium channel blockers are used to treat hypertension.
Diazepam	Diazepam , first marketed as Valium by Hoffmann-La Roche, is a benzodiazepine derivative drug. It is commonly used for treating anxiety, insomnia, seizures, muscle spasms, restless legs syndrome, alcohol withdrawal, benzodiazepine withdrawal, and Ménière's disease. It may also be used before certain medical procedures to reduce tension and anxiety, and in some surgical procedures to induce amnesia.
Endorphin	Endorphins are endogenous opioid polypeptide compounds. They are produced by the pituitary gland and the hypothalamus in vertebrates during strenuous exercise, excitement, pain, consumption of spicy food and orgasm, and they resemble the opiates in their abilities to produce analgesia and a feeling of well-being. Endorphins work as 'natural pain relievers.' The term 'Endorphin' implies a pharmacological activity (analogous to the activity of the corticosteroid category of biochemicals) as opposed to a specific chemical formulation.
Fluoxetine	Fluoxetine (trade name Prozac) is an antidepressant of the selective serotonin reuptake inhibitor (SSRI) class. Fluoxetine is approved for the treatment of major depression (including pediatric depression), obsessive-compulsive disorder (in both adult and pediatric populations), bulimia nervosa, anorexia nervosa, panic disorder and premenstrual dysphoric disorder. Despite the availability of newer agents, it remains extremely popular.
Norepinephrine	Noradrenaline (BAN) is a catecholamine with dual roles as a hormone and a neurotransmitter.

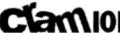

Chapter 3. Signal Transduction and the Chemically Addressed Nervous System

	As a stress hormone, Norepinephrine affects parts of the brain where attention and responding actions are controlled. Along with epinephrine, Norepinephrine also underlies the fight-or-flight response, directly increasing heart rate, triggering the release of glucose from energy stores, and increasing blood flow to skeletal muscle.
Pharmacology	Pharmacology is the study of drug action. More specifically, it is the study of the interactions that occur between a living organism and exogenous chemicals that alter normal biochemical function. If substances have medicinal properties, they are considered pharmaceuticals.
Abuse	Abuse is defined as:
Cocaine	Cocaine is a crystalline tropane alkaloid that is obtained from the leaves of the coca plant. The name comes from 'coca' in addition to the alkaloid suffix -ine, forming Cocaine. It is a stimulant of the central nervous system and an appetite suppressant.
Aventyl	Nortriptyline is a second-generation tricyclic antidepressant marketed as the hydrochloride under the trade names Sensoval, Aventyl, Pamelor, Norpress, Allegron and Nortrilen. It is used in the treatment of major depression and childhood nocturnal enuresis (bedwetting). In addition, it is sometimes used for chronic illnesses such as chronic fatigue syndrome, chronic pain and migraines, and labile affect in some neurological conditions.
Pamelor	Nortriptyline is a second-generation tricyclic antidepressant marketed as the hydrochloride under the trade names Sensoval, Aventyl, Pamelor, Norpress, Allegron and Nortrilen. It is used in the treatment of major depression and childhood nocturnal enuresis (bedwetting). In addition, it is sometimes used for chronic illnesses such as chronic fatigue syndrome, chronic pain and migraines, and labile affect in some neurological conditions.
Nortriptyline	Nortriptyline is a second-generation tricyclic antidepressant marketed as the hydrochloride under the trade names Sensoval, Aventyl, Pamelor, Norpress, Allegron and Nortrilen. It is used in the treatment of major depression and childhood nocturnal enuresis (bedwetting). In addition, it is sometimes used for chronic illnesses such as chronic fatigue syndrome, chronic pain and migraines, and labile affect in some neurological conditions.
Bipolar disorder	Bipolar disorder or manic-depressive disorder is a psychiatric diagnosis that describes a category of mood disorders defined by the presence of one or more episodes of abnormally elevated mood clinically referred to as mania or, if milder, hypomania. Individuals who experience manic episodes also commonly experience depressive episodes or symptoms, or mixed episodes in which features of both mania and depression are present at the same time. These episodes are usually separated by periods of 'normal' mood, but in some individuals, depression and mania may rapidly alternate, known as rapid cycling.

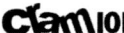

Chapter 3. Signal Transduction and the Chemically Addressed Nervous System

Huntington's disease	Huntington's disease is a neurodegenerative genetic disorder that affects muscle coordination and leads to cognitive decline and dementia. It typically becomes noticeable in middle age. Huntington's disease is the most common genetic cause of abnormal involuntary writhing movements called chorea.
Dopamine	Dopamine is a neurotransmitter that occurs in a wide variety of animals, including both vertebrates and invertebrates. In the brain, this phenethylamine functions as a neurotransmitter, activating the five types of Dopamine receptors--D_1, D_2, D_3, D_4, and D_5--and their variants. Dopamine is produced in several areas of the brain, including the substantia nigra and the ventral tegmental area.
Schizophrenia	Schizophrenia , from the Greek roots skhizein and phrÄ"n, phren- (φρÎ®ν, φρεν-; 'mind') is a psychiatric diagnosis that describes a neuropsychiatric and mental disorder characterized by abnormalities in the perception or expression of reality. It most commonly manifests as auditory hallucinations, paranoid or bizarre delusions, or disorganized speech and thinking with significant social or occupational dysfunction. Onset of symptoms typically occurs in young adulthood, with around 0.4-0.6% of the population affected.
Molindone	Molindone is a therapeutic antipsychotic, used in the treatment of schizophrenia. It works by blocking the effects of dopamine in the brain, leading to diminished psychoses. It is rapidly absorbed when taken by mouth.
Sodium	Sodium is a metallic element with a symbol Na and atomic number 11. It is a soft, silvery-white, highly reactive metal and is a member of the alkali metals within 'group 1' (formerly known as 'group IA'). It has only one stable isotope, ^{23}Na.
Sodium channel	Sodium channels are integral membrane proteins that form ion channels, conducting sodium ions (Na^+) through a cell's plasma membrane. They are classified according to the trigger that opens the channel for such ions, i.e. either a voltage-change (voltage-gated Sodium channels) or binding of a substance (a ligand) to the channel (ligand-gated Sodium channels). In excitable cells such as neurons, myocytes, and certain types of glia, Sodium channels are responsible for the rising phase of action potentials.
Enzyme	Enzymes are proteins that catalyze (i.e., increase the rates of) chemical reactions. In enzymatic reactions, the molecules at the beginning of the process are called substrates, and the Enzyme converts them into different molecules, called the products. Almost all processes in a biological cell need Enzymes to occur at significant rates.

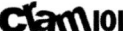

Chapter 3. Signal Transduction and the Chemically Addressed Nervous System

Phosphatase	A Phosphatase is an enzyme that removes a phosphate group from its substrate by hydrolysing phosphoric acid monoesters into a phosphate ion and a molecule with a free hydroxyl group . This action is directly opposite to that of phosphorylases and kinases, which attach phosphate groups to their substrates by using energetic molecules like ATP. A common Phosphatase in many organisms is alkaline Phosphatase.
	Protein phosphorylation is the most common and important form of reversible protein posttranslational modification (PTM), with up to 30% of all proteins being phosphorylated at any given time.
Antihistamine	A histamine antagonist is an agent that serves to inhibit the release or action of histamine. antihistamine can be used to describe any histamine antagonist, but it is usually reserved for the classical antihistamines that act upon the H_1 histamine receptor.
	antihistamines are used as treatment for allergies.
Histidine	Histidine Histidine an essential amino acid, has a positively charged imidazole functional group. It is the one of the 22 proteinogenic amino acids. Its codons are CAU and CAC. Histidine was first isolated by German physician Albrecht Kossel in 1896. Histidine is an essential amino acid in humans and other mammals.
Superfamily	The term Superfamily is used to describe several different concepts in different scientific fields:
	· Taxonomic rank: Superfamily is a level of biological classification
	· Superfamily: in comparative linguistics, another term for 'macrofamily'
	· Superfamily: in molecular biology, a large group of related proteins or other molecules.
	· Superfamily: a Norwegian pop band
	· Superfamily: database of annotation for all proteins
Hormone	A hormone is a chemical released by one or more cells that affects cells in other parts of the organism. Only a small amount of hormone is required to alter cell metabolism. It is essentially a chemical messenger that transports a signal from one cell to another.

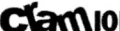

Chapter 3. Signal Transduction and the Chemically Addressed Nervous System

Tyrosine	Tyrosine or 4-hydroxyphenylalanine, is one of the 20 amino acids that are used by cells to synthesize proteins. It is a non-essential amino acid with a polar side group. The word 'Tyrosine' is from the Greek tyros, meaning cheese, as it was first discovered in 1846 by German chemist Justus von Liebig in the protein casein from cheese.
Adenosine	Adenosine is a nucleoside composed of a molecule of adenine attached to a ribose sugar molecule (ribofuranose) moiety via a β-N_9-glycosidic bond. Adenosine plays an important role in biochemical processes, such as energy transfer--as Adenosine triphosphate (ATP) and Adenosine diphosphate (ADP)--as well as in signal transduction as cyclic Adenosine monophosphate, cAMP. It is also an inhibitory neurotransmitter, believed to play a role in promoting sleep and suppressing arousal, with levels increasing with each hour an organism is awake. Adenosine is often abbreviated Ado.
Prolixin	Fluphenazine is a typical antipsychotic drug used for the treatment of psychoses such as schizophrenia and acute manic phases of bipolar disorder. It belongs to the piperazine class of phenothiazines and is extremely potent; more potent than haloperidol and around fifty to seventy times the potency of chlorpromazine. It is marketed under the brand name of Prolixin and Sydocate(Surge Laboratories).
Calcineurin	Calcineurin is a protein phosphatase also known as protein phosphatase 3, PPP3CA, and formerly known as protein phosphatase 2B (PP2B). It activates the T cells of the immune system and can be blocked by drugs. Calcineurin activates NFATc (Nuclear Factor of Activated T cell, cytoplasmic), a transcription factor by dephosphorylating it.
Valproate semisodium	Valproate semisodium or divalproex sodium (USAN) consists of a compound of sodium valproate and valproic acid in a 1:1 molar relationship in an enteric coated form. It is used in the UK, Canada, and U.S. for the treatment of the manic episodes of bipolar disorder. In rare cases, it is also used as a treatment for major depressive disorder, and increasingly taken long-term for prevention of both manic and depressive phases of bipolar disorder, especially the rapid-cycling variant.
Phosphorylation	Phosphorylation is the addition of a phosphate (PO_4^{3-}) group to a protein or other organic molecule. Phosphorylation activates or deactivates many protein enzymes.

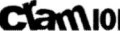

	Protein phosphorylation in particular plays a significant role in a wide range of cellular processes.
MAOIs	Monoamine oxidase inhibitors (MAOIs) are a class of powerful antidepressant drugs prescribed for the treatment of depression. They are particularly effective in treating atypical depression, and have also shown efficacy in smoking cessation.
	Due to potentially lethal dietary and drug interactions, MAOIs had been reserved as a last line of defense, used only when other classes of antidepressant drugs (for example selective serotonin reuptake inhibitors and tricyclic antidepressants) have failed.
Hypertension	Hypertension is a chronic medical condition in which the blood pressure is elevated. It is also referred to as high blood pressure or shortened to HT, HTN or HPN. The word 'Hypertension', by itself, normally refers to systemic, arterial Hypertension.
	Hypertension can be classified as either essential (primary) or secondary.
Protein kinase	A Protein kinase is a kinase enzyme that modifies other proteins by chemically adding phosphate groups to them (phosphorylation). Phosphorylation usually results in a functional change of the target protein (substrate) by changing enzyme activity, cellular location, or association with other proteins. The human genome contains about 500 Protein kinase genes and they constitute about 2% of all human genes.
Neurotrophin	Neurotrophins are a family of proteins that induce the survival, development, and function of neurons.
	They belong to a class of growth factors, secreted proteins that are capable of signaling particular cells to survive, differentiate, or grow. Growth factors such as neurotrophins that promote the survival of neurons are known as neurotrophic factors.
Iloperidone	Iloperidone is an atypical antipsychotic for the treatment of schizophrenia. It was approved by the U.S. Food and Drug Administration (FDA) for use in the United States on May 6, 2009.

Chapter 3. Signal Transduction and the Chemically Addressed Nervous System

Imipramine	Imipramine is an antidepressant medication, a tricyclic antidepressant of the dibenzazepine group. Imipramine is mainly used in the treatment of major depression and enuresis (inability to control urination). It has also been evaluated for use in panic disorder.
Syndrome	In medicine and psychology, a Syndrome is the association of several clinically recognizable features, signs (observed by a physician), symptoms (reported by the patient), phenomena or characteristics that often occur together, so that the presence of one feature alerts the physician to the presence of the others. In recent decades, the term has been used outside medicine to refer to a combination of phenomena seen in association. The term Syndrome derives from its Greek roots and means literally 'run together', as the features do.

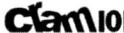

Chapter 4. Transporters and G Protein Linked Receptors

Symptom	A Symptom is a departure from normal function or feeling which is noticed by a patient, indicating the presence of disease or abnormality. A Symptom is subjective, observed by the patient, and not measured.
Neurotransmitters	Neurotransmitters are endogenous chemicals which relay, amplify, and modulate signals between a neuron and another cell. Neurotransmitters are packaged into synaptic vesicles that cluster beneath the membrane on the presynaptic side of a synapse, and are released into the synaptic cleft, where they bind to receptors in the membrane on the postsynaptic side of the synapse. Release of Neurotransmitters usually follows arrival of an action potential at the synapse, but may follow graded electrical potentials.
Sinequan	Doxepin is a psychotropic agent with tricyclic antidepressant and anxiolytic properties, known under many brand-names such as Aponal, the original preparation by Boehringer-Mannheim, now part of the Roche group; Adapine, Deptran, Sinquan and Sinequan . As doxepin hydrochloride, it is the active ingredient in cream-based preparations (Zonalon and Xepin) for the treatment of dermatological itch. Doxepin is currently investigated for the treatment of insomnia, and the proposed tradename of doxepin for this indication is Silenor.
Amyloid	Amyloids are insoluble fibrous protein aggregates sharing specific structural traits. Abnormal accumulation of amyloid in organs may lead to amyloidosis, and may play a role in various neurodegenerative diseases. The name amyloid comes from the early mistaken identification of the substance as starch, based on crude iodine-staining techniques.
Dopamine	Dopamine is a neurotransmitter that occurs in a wide variety of animals, including both vertebrates and invertebrates. In the brain, this phenethylamine functions as a neurotransmitter, activating the five types of Dopamine receptors--D_1, D_2, D_3, D_4, and D_5--and their variants. Dopamine is produced in several areas of the brain, including the substantia nigra and the ventral tegmental area.
Mirtazapine	Mirtazapine is a psychoactive drug of the benzazepine and tetracyclic antidepressant (TeCA) chemical classes which is used primarily as an antidepressant. It is sometimes used for its anxiolytic, hypnotic, antiemetic, orexigenic, and antihistamine or antipruritic effects. Mirtazapine was introduced by Organon International in 1994. Along with its chemical analogue and predecessor mianserin (Bolvidon, Norval, Tolvon), Mirtazapine is one of the few noradrenergic and specific serotonergic antidepressants (NaSSAs).

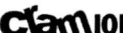

Chapter 4. Transporters and G Protein Linked Receptors

Norepinephrine	Noradrenaline (BAN) is a catecholamine with dual roles as a hormone and a neurotransmitter. As a stress hormone, Norepinephrine affects parts of the brain where attention and responding actions are controlled. Along with epinephrine, Norepinephrine also underlies the fight-or-flight response, directly increasing heart rate, triggering the release of glucose from energy stores, and increasing blood flow to skeletal muscle.
Receptor	In biochemistry, a receptor is a protein molecule, embedded in either the plasma membrane or the cytoplasm of a cell, to which one or more specific kinds of signaling molecules may attach. A molecule which binds (attaches) to a receptor is called a ligand, and may be a peptide (short protein) or other small molecule, such as a neurotransmitter, a hormone, a pharmaceutical drug, or a toxin. Each kind of receptor can bind only certain ligand shapes.
Serotonin	Serotonin is a monoamine neurotransmitter. Biochemically derived from tryptophan, serotonin is primarily found in the gastrointestinal (GI) tract, platelets, and in the central nervous system (CNS) of animals including humans. It is a well-known contributor to feelings of well-being; therefore it is also known as a 'happiness hormone' despite not being a hormone.
Abuse	Abuse is defined as:
Acetylcholine	The chemical compound Acetylcholine is a neurotransmitter in both the peripheral nervous system (PNS) and central nervous system (CNS) in many organisms including humans. Acetylcholine is one of many neurotransmitters in the autonomic nervous system (ANS) and the only neurotransmitter used in the motor division of the somatic nervous system. (Sensory neurons use glutamate and various peptides at their synapses).
Amphetamine	Amphetamine (amfetamine (INN)) is a psychostimulant drug that is known to produce increased wakefulness and focus in association with decreased fatigue and appetite. Amphetamine is related to drugs such as methAmphetamine and dextroAmphetamine, which are a group of potent drugs that act by increasing levels of dopamine and norepinephrine in the brain, inducing euphoria. The group includes prescription CNS drugs commonly used to treat attention-deficit hyperactivity disorder (ADHD).
Cocaine	Cocaine is a crystalline tropane alkaloid that is obtained from the leaves of the coca plant. The name comes from 'coca' in addition to the alkaloid suffix -ine, forming Cocaine. It is a stimulant of the central nervous system and an appetite suppressant.

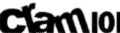

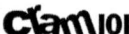

Adenosine	Adenosine is a nucleoside composed of a molecule of adenine attached to a ribose sugar molecule (ribofuranose) moiety via a β-N_9-glycosidic bond.
	Adenosine plays an important role in biochemical processes, such as energy transfer--as Adenosine triphosphate (ATP) and Adenosine diphosphate (ADP)--as well as in signal transduction as cyclic Adenosine monophosphate, cAMP. It is also an inhibitory neurotransmitter, believed to play a role in promoting sleep and suppressing arousal, with levels increasing with each hour an organism is awake.
	Adenosine is often abbreviated Ado.
Potassium	Potassium is the chemical element with the symbol K , atomic number 19, and atomic mass 39.0983. Potassium was first isolated from potash. Elemental Potassium is a soft silvery-white metallic alkali metal that oxidizes rapidly in air and is very reactive with water, generating sufficient heat to ignite the evolved hydrogen.
Sodium	Sodium is a metallic element with a symbol Na and atomic number 11. It is a soft, silvery-white, highly reactive metal and is a member of the alkali metals within 'group 1' (formerly known as 'group IA'). It has only one stable isotope, ^{23}Na.
Antidepressant	An antidepressant is a psychiatric medication used to alleviate mood disorders, such as major depression and dysthymia and anxiety disorders such as social anxiety disorder. According to Gelder, Mayou '*Geddes (2005) people with a depressive illness will experience a therapeutic effect to their mood, however this will not be experienced in healthy individuals. Drugs including the monoamine oxidase inhibitors (MAOIs), tricyclic antidepressants (TCAs), tetracyclic antidepressants (TeCAs), selective serotonin reuptake inhibitors (SSRIs), and serotonin-norepinephrine reuptake inhibitors (SNRIs) are most commonly associated with the term.
Psychopharmacology	Psychopharmacology is the study of drug-induced changes in mood, sensation, thinking, and behavior.
	The field of Psychopharmacology studies a wide range of substances with various types of psychoactive properties. The professional and commercial fields of pharmacology and Psychopharmacology do not mainly focus on psychedelic or recreational drugs, as the majority of studies are conducted for the development, study, and use of drugs for the modification of behavior and the alleviation of symptoms, particularly in the treatment of mental disorders .

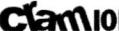

53

Chapter 4. Transporters and G Protein Linked Receptors

Amino acid	Amino acids are molecules containing an amine group, a carboxylic acid group and a side-chain that varies between different amino acids. The key elements of an amino acid are carbon, hydrogen, oxygen, and nitrogen. They are particularly important in biochemistry, where the term usually refers to alpha-amino acids.
Tiagabine	Tiagabine is an anti-convulsive medication produced by Cephalon and marketed under the brand name Gabitril. The drug was discovered at Novo Nordisk in Denmark in 1988 and was co-developed with Abbott. After a period of co-promotion, Cephalon licensed Tiagabine from Abbott/Novo and now is the exclusive producer. It is believed that the pharmacology is related to its ability, documented in in vitro experiments, to enhance the activity of gamma aminobutyric acid (GABA), the major inhibitory neurotransmitter in the central nervous system. These experiments have shown that Tiagabine binds to recognition sites associated with the GABA uptake carrier. It is thought that, by this action, Tiagabine blocks GABA uptake into presynaptic neurons, permitting more GABA to be available for receptor binding on the surfaces of post-synaptic cells. Evidence is available that it operates as a selective GABA reuptake inhibitor.
Trifluoperazine	Trifluoperazine is a typical antipsychotic drug of the phenothiazine group. Trifluoperazine has central antiadrenergic, antidopaminergic, and minimal anticholinergic effects. It is believed to work by blockading dopamine D_1 and D_2 receptors in the mesocortical and mesolimbic pathways, relieving or minimizing such symptoms of schizophrenia as hallucinations, delusions, and disorganized thought and speech.
Antipsychotic	An antipsychotic is a tranquilizing psychiatric medication primarily used to manage psychosis (including delusions or hallucinations, as well as disordered thought), particularly in schizophrenia and bipolar disorder. A first generation of antipsychotics, known as typical antipsychotics, was discovered in the 1950s. Most of the drugs in the second generation, known as atypical antipsychotics, have been developed more recently, although the first atypical antipsychotic, clozapine, was discovered in the 1950s and introduced clinically in the 1970s.
Atypical antipsychotics	The Atypical antipsychotics are a group of antipsychotic drugs used to treat psychiatric conditions. Some Atypical antipsychotics are FDA approved for use in the treatment of schizophrenia. Some carry FDA approved indications for acute mania, bipolar mania, psychotic agitation, bipolar maintenance, and other indications.
Triglycerides	(more properly known as , TAG or triacylglyceride) is a glyceride in which the glycerol is esterified with three fatty acids. It is the main constituent of vegetable oil and animal fats.

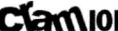

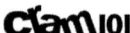

Chapter 4. Transporters and G Protein Linked Receptors

	Triglycerides are formed from a single molecule of glycerol, combined with three fatty acids on each of the OH groups, and make up most of fats digested by humans.
Folinic acid	Folinic acid or leucovorin (USAN), generally administered as calcium or sodium folinate (or leucovorin calcium/sodium), is an adjuvant used in cancer chemotherapy involving the drug methotrexate. It is also used in synergistic combination with the chemotherapy agent 5-fluorouracil. LevoFolinic acid and its salts are the enantiopure drugs.
Levetiracetam	Levetiracetam (INN) is an anticonvulsant medication used to treat epilepsy. It is S-enantiomer of etiracetam, structurally similar to the prototypical nootropic drug piracetam. Levetiracetam is marketed under the trade name Keppra.
Atrophy	Atrophy is the partial or complete wasting away of a part of the body. Causes of Atrophy include poor nourishment, poor circulation, loss of hormonal support, loss of nerve supply to the target organ, disuse or lack of exercise or disease intrinsic to the tissue itself. Hormonal and nerve inputs that maintain an organ or body part are referred to as trophic [noun] in medical practice.
Glucocorticoid	Glucocorticoids (GC) are a class of steroid hormones that bind to the Glucocorticoid receptor (GR), which is present in almost every vertebrate animal cell. The name Glucocorticoid derives from their role in the regulation of the metabolism of glucose, their synthesis in the adrenal cortex, and their steroidal structure . GCs are part of the feedback mechanism in the immune system that turns immune activity (inflammation) down.
Seizure	An epileptic Seizure is a transient symptom of excessive or synchronous neuronal activity in the brain. It can manifest as an alteration in mental state, tonic or clonic movements, convulsions, and various other psychic symptoms (such as déjà vu or jamais vu). The medical syndrome of recurrent, unprovoked Seizures is termed epilepsy, but Seizures can occur in people who do not have epilepsy.
Bupropion	Bupropion previously known as amfebutamone, is an atypical antidepressant and smoking cessation aid. It acts as a strong norepinephrine and weak dopamine reuptake inhibitor, as well as $\alpha_3\beta_4$-nicotinic receptor antagonist. Bupropion belongs to the chemical class of aminoketones and is similar in structure to cathinone and diethylpropion, and to phenethylamines in general.

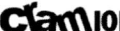

Chapter 4. Transporters and G Protein☐Linked Receptors

Galantamine	Galantamine is a chemical used for the treatment of mild to moderate Alzheimer's disease and various memory impairments. It is an alkaloid that is obtained synthetically or from the bulbs and flowers of the Caucasian snowdrop (Voronov's snowdrop), Galanthus woronowii (Amaryllidaceae) and related genera like Narcissus (daffodil), Leucojum (snowflake) and Lycoris including Lycoris radiata (Red Spider Lily). The active ingredient was isolated by prof.
Mechanism of action	In pharmacology, the term Mechanism of action refers to the specific biochemical interaction through which a drug substance produces its pharmacological effect. A Mechanism of action usually includes mention of the specific molecular targets to which the drug binds, such as an enzyme or receptor.
	For example, the Mechanism of action of aspirin involves irreversible inhibition of the enzyme cyclooxygenase, which suppresses the production of prostaglandins and thromboxanes, thereby reducing pain and inflammation.
Methylphenidate	Methylphenidate is a psychostimulant drug approved for treatment of attention-deficit hyperactivity disorder, Postural Orthostatic Tachycardia Syndrome and narcolepsy. It may also be prescribed for off-label use in treatment-resistant cases of lethargy, depression, neural insult, and obesity. Methylphenidate belongs to the piperidine class of compounds and increases the levels of dopamine and norepinephrine in the brain through reuptake inhibition of the monoamine transporters.
Tianeptine	Tianeptine is a selective serotonin reuptake enhancer (SSRE) drug used for treating Major depressive episodes (mild, moderate, or severe). Unlike conventional tricyclic antidepressants, Tianeptine enhances the reuptake of serotonin instead of inhibiting it, opposite to the action of SSRIs. Moreover, it enhances the extracellular concentration of dopamine in the nucleus accumbens.
Interaction	Interaction is a kind of action that occurs as two or more objects have an effect upon one another. The idea of a two-way effect is essential in the concept of Interaction, as opposed to a one-way causal effect. A closely related term is interconnectivity, which deals with the Interactions of Interactions within systems: combinations of many simple Interactions can lead to surprising emergent phenomena.

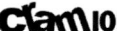

Chapter 4. Transporters and G Protein□Linked Receptors

Schizophrenia	Schizophrenia , from the Greek roots skhizein and phrÄ"n, phren- (φρÎ®v, φρεν-; 'mind') is a psychiatric diagnosis that describes a neuropsychiatric and mental disorder characterized by abnormalities in the perception or expression of reality. It most commonly manifests as auditory hallucinations, paranoid or bizarre delusions, or disorganized speech and thinking with significant social or occupational dysfunction. Onset of symptoms typically occurs in young adulthood, with around 0.4-0.6% of the population affected.
Action of drugs	The action of drugs on the human body is called pharmacodynamics, and what the body does with the drug is called pharmacokinetics. The drugs that enter the human tend to stimulate certain receptors, ion channels, act on enzymes or transporter proteins. As a result, they cause the human body to react in a specific way.
Agonist	An Agonist is a drug that binds to a receptor of a cell and triggers a response by the cell. An Agonist often mimics the action of a naturally occurring substance. An Agonist produces an action.
Constitutive	The term 'Constitutive' might refer to: · In physics, a Constitutive equation is a relation between two physical quantities · In cell biology, a Constitutively active protein is a protein whose activity is constant and active · In ecology, a Constitutive defense is one which is always active, as opposed to an inducible defense. · Constitutive theory of statehood · In genetics, Constitutive refers to a gene product made all the time. Ie. In the absence of the activator or the repressor, RNA polymerase transcribes the gene Constitutively.
Acetylcholinesterase	Acetylcholinesterase is an enzyme that degrades (through its hydrolytic activity) the neurotransmitter acetylcholine, producing choline and an acetate group. It is mainly found at neuromuscular junctions and cholinergic nervous system, where its activity serves to terminate synaptic transmission. Acetylcholinesterase has a very high catalytic activity -- each molecule of Acetylcholinesterase degrades about 25000 molecules of acetylcholine per second.

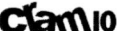

Chapter 4. Transporters and G Protein☐Linked Receptors

Half-life	Half-life is the period of time it takes for a substance undergoing decay to decrease by half. The name was originally used to describe a characteristic of unstable atoms (radioactive decay), but may apply to any quantity which follows a set-rate decay. The original term, dating to 1907, was 'Half-life period', which was later shortened to 'Half-life' in the early 1950s.
Monoamine oxidase	L-Monoamine oxidases (MAO) (EC 1.4.3.4) are a family of enzymes that catalyze the oxidation of monoamines. They are found bound to the outer membrane of mitochondria in most cell types in the body. The enzyme was originally discovered by Mary Bernheim (née Hare) in the liver and was named tyramine oxidase.
Melatonin	Melatonin , also known chemically as N-acetyl-5-methoxytryptamine, is a naturally occurring compound found in animals, plants, and microbes. In animals, circulating levels of Melatonin vary in a daily cycle, thereby regulating the circadian rhythms of several biological functions. Many biological effects of Melatonin are produced through activation of Melatonin receptors, while others are due to its role as a pervasive and powerful antioxidant, with a particular role in the protection of nuclear and mitochondrial DNA. Melatonin in plants has multiple roles, including regulation of the photoperiod, in plant defence responses, and as a scavenger of reactive oxygen species.
Histamine	Histamine is a biogenic amine involved in local immune responses as well as regulating physiological function in the gut and acting as a neurotransmitter. Histamine triggers the inflammatory response. As part of an immune response to foreign pathogens, Histamine is produced by basophils and by mast cells found in nearby connective tissues.
Inverse agonist	In pharmacology, an Inverse agonist is an agent which binds to the same receptor binding-site as an agonist for that receptor and reverses constitutive activity of receptors. Inverse agonists exert the opposite pharmacological effect of a receptor agonist. Inverse agonists are effective against certain types of receptors (e.g. certain histamine receptors and GABA receptors) which have intrinsic activity without the action of a ligand upon them (also referred to as 'constitutive activity').

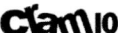

Chapter 5. Ion Channels and Enzymes Targets of Psychopharmacological Drug Action

Lewy bodies	Lewy bodies are abnormal aggregates of protein that develop inside nerve cells in Parkinson's disease (PD) and some other disorders. They are identified under the microscope when histology is performed on the brain. Lewy bodies appear as spherical masses that displace other cell components.
Cholinergic	A receptor is cholinergic if it uses acetylcholine as its neurotransmitter. cholinergic means related to the neurotransmitter acetylcholine, and is typically used in a neurological perspective. The parasympathetic nervous system is entirely cholinergic.
Receptor	In biochemistry, a receptor is a protein molecule, embedded in either the plasma membrane or the cytoplasm of a cell, to which one or more specific kinds of signaling molecules may attach. A molecule which binds (attaches) to a receptor is called a ligand, and may be a peptide (short protein) or other small molecule, such as a neurotransmitter, a hormone, a pharmaceutical drug, or a toxin. Each kind of receptor can bind only certain ligand shapes.
Symptom	A Symptom is a departure from normal function or feeling which is noticed by a patient, indicating the presence of disease or abnormality. A Symptom is subjective, observed by the patient, and not measured.
Prolixin	Fluphenazine is a typical antipsychotic drug used for the treatment of psychoses such as schizophrenia and acute manic phases of bipolar disorder. It belongs to the piperazine class of phenothiazines and is extremely potent; more potent than haloperidol and around fifty to seventy times the potency of chlorpromazine. It is marketed under the brand name of Prolixin and Sydocate(Surge Laboratories).
Amyloid	Amyloids are insoluble fibrous protein aggregates sharing specific structural traits. Abnormal accumulation of amyloid in organs may lead to amyloidosis, and may play a role in various neurodegenerative diseases. The name amyloid comes from the early mistaken identification of the substance as starch, based on crude iodine-staining techniques.

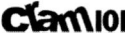

Chapter 5. Ion Channels and Enzymes Targets of Psychopharmacological Drug Action

Calcium	Calcium is the chemical element with the symbol Ca and atomic number 20. It has an atomic mass of 40.078 amu. Calcium is a soft gray alkaline earth metal, and is the fifth most abundant element by mass in the Earth's crust. Calcium is also the fifth most abundant dissolved ion in seawater by both molarity and mass, after sodium, chloride, magnesium, and sulfate.
Calcium channel	A Calcium channel is an ion channel which displays selective permeabiltiy to calcium ions. It is sometimes synonymous as voltage-dependent Calcium channel, although there are also ligand-gated Calcium channels. The following tables explain gating, gene, location and function of different types of Calcium channels, both voltage and ligand-gated. · the receptor-operated Calcium channels (in vasoconstriction) · P2X receptor Calcium channel blockers are used to treat hypertension.
Pharmacology	Pharmacology is the study of drug action. More specifically, it is the study of the interactions that occur between a living organism and exogenous chemicals that alter normal biochemical function. If substances have medicinal properties, they are considered pharmaceuticals.
Prolactin	Prolactin or Luteotropic hormone (LTH) is a peptide hormone discovered by Dr. Henry Friesen, primarily associated with lactation. In breastfeeding, the act of an infant suckling the nipple stimulates the production of Prolactin, which fills the breast with milk via a process called lactogenesis, in preparation for the next feed. Oxytocin, another hormone, is also released, which triggers milk let-down.
Transdermal	Transdermal is a route of administration wherein active ingredients are delivered across the skin for systemic distribution. Examples include Transdermal patches used for medicine delivery, and Transdermal implants used for medical or aesthetic purposes. Although the skin is a large and logical target for drug delivery, its basic functions limit its utility for this purpose.

CᒪᗩᗰﾉO/

Chapter 5. Ion Channels and Enzymes Targets of Psychopharmacological Drug Action

Glutamate receptors	Glutamate receptors are synaptic receptors located primarily on the membranes of neuronal cells. Glutamate is one of the 20 amino acids used to assemble proteins and as a result is abundant in many areas of the body, but it also functions as a neurotransmitter and is particularly abundant in the nervous system. Glutamate receptors are responsible for the glutamate-mediated post-synaptic excitation of neural cells, and are important for neural communication, memory formation, learning, and regulation.
Agonist	An Agonist is a drug that binds to a receptor of a cell and triggers a response by the cell. An Agonist often mimics the action of a naturally occurring substance. An Agonist produces an action.
Opioid	An opioid is a chemical that works by binding to opioid receptors, which are found principally in the central nervous system and the gastrointestinal tract. The receptors in these two organ systems mediate both the beneficial effects and the side effects of opioids. The analgesic effects of opioids are due to decreased perception of pain, decreased reaction to pain as well as increased pain tolerance.
Peptide	Peptides are short polymers formed from the linking, in a defined order, of α-amino acids. The link between one amino acid residue and the next is called an amide bond or a Peptide bond. Proteins are polyPeptide molecules, or consist of multiple polyPeptide subunits, each composed of chains containing a specific sequence of the 22 proteinogenic amino acids.
Sodium	Sodium is a metallic element with a symbol Na and atomic number 11. It is a soft, silvery-white, highly reactive metal and is a member of the alkali metals within 'group 1' (formerly known as 'group IA'). It has only one stable isotope, ^{23}Na.
Sodium channel	Sodium channels are integral membrane proteins that form ion channels, conducting sodium ions (Na^+) through a cell's plasma membrane. They are classified according to the trigger that opens the channel for such ions, i.e. either a voltage-change (voltage-gated Sodium channels) or binding of a substance (a ligand) to the channel (ligand-gated Sodium channels). In excitable cells such as neurons, myocytes, and certain types of glia, Sodium channels are responsible for the rising phase of action potentials.

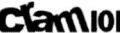

Chapter 5. Ion Channels and Enzymes Targets of Psychopharmacological Drug Action

Acetylcholine	The chemical compound Acetylcholine is a neurotransmitter in both the peripheral nervous system (PNS) and central nervous system (CNS) in many organisms including humans. Acetylcholine is one of many neurotransmitters in the autonomic nervous system (ANS) and the only neurotransmitter used in the motor division of the somatic nervous system. (Sensory neurons use glutamate and various peptides at their synapses).
Benadryl	Benadryl is a brand name allergy medicine marketed over-the-counter by Johnson ' Johnson subsidiary McNeil Consumer Healthcare. Prior to 2007, Benadryl was marketed by Pfizer Consumer Healthcare. Benadryl is used as an antihistamine for the temporary relief of seasonal and perennial allergy symptoms.
Antipsychotic	An antipsychotic is a tranquilizing psychiatric medication primarily used to manage psychosis (including delusions or hallucinations, as well as disordered thought), particularly in schizophrenia and bipolar disorder. A first generation of antipsychotics, known as typical antipsychotics, was discovered in the 1950s. Most of the drugs in the second generation, known as atypical antipsychotics, have been developed more recently, although the first atypical antipsychotic, clozapine, was discovered in the 1950s and introduced clinically in the 1970s.
Inverse agonist	In pharmacology, an Inverse agonist is an agent which binds to the same receptor binding-site as an agonist for that receptor and reverses constitutive activity of receptors. Inverse agonists exert the opposite pharmacological effect of a receptor agonist. Inverse agonists are effective against certain types of receptors (e.g. certain histamine receptors and GABA receptors) which have intrinsic activity without the action of a ligand upon them (also referred to as 'constitutive activity').
Magnesium	All forms of life require magnesium, and yet the molecular mechanisms of Mg^{2+} uptake from the environment and the distribution (transport) of this vital element within the organism are only slowly being elucidated. In bacteria Mg^{2+} is probably mainly supplied by the CorA protein and, where the CorA protein is absent, by the MgtE protein. In yeast the initial uptake is via the Alr1p and Alr2p proteins, but at this stage the only internal Mg^{2+} distributing protein identified is Mrs2p.
Excitotoxicity	Excitotoxicity is the pathological process by which nerve cells are damaged and killed by glutamate and similar substances. This occurs when receptors for the excitatory neurotransmitter glutamate (glutamate receptors) such as the NMDA receptor and AMPA receptor are overactivated. Excitotoxins like NMDA and kainic acid which bind to these receptors, as well as pathologically high levels of glutamate, can cause Excitotoxicity by allowing high levels of calcium ions (Ca^{2+}) to enter the cell.

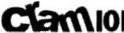

Chapter 5. Ion Channels and Enzymes Targets of Psychopharmacological Drug Action

Long-term potentiation	In neuroscience, Long-term potentiation is a long-lasting enhancement in signal transmission between two neurons that results from stimulating them synchronously. It is one of several phenomena underlying synaptic plasticity, the ability of chemical synapses to change their strength. As memories are thought to be encoded by modification of synaptic strength, LTP is widely considered one of the major cellular mechanisms that underlies learning and memory.
Phencyclidine	Phencyclidine, commonly initialized as PCP, is a recreational dissociative drug. Formerly used as an anesthetic agent, PCP exhibits both hallucinogenic and neurotoxic effects.
Potassium	Potassium is the chemical element with the symbol K , atomic number 19, and atomic mass 39.0983. Potassium was first isolated from potash. Elemental Potassium is a soft silvery-white metallic alkali metal that oxidizes rapidly in air and is very reactive with water, generating sufficient heat to ignite the evolved hydrogen.
Syndrome	In medicine and psychology, a Syndrome is the association of several clinically recognizable features, signs (observed by a physician), symptoms (reported by the patient), phenomena or characteristics that often occur together, so that the presence of one feature alerts the physician to the presence of the others. In recent decades, the term has been used outside medicine to refer to a combination of phenomena seen in association. The term Syndrome derives from its Greek roots and means literally 'run together', as the features do.
Valproate semisodium	Valproate semisodium or divalproex sodium (USAN) consists of a compound of sodium valproate and valproic acid in a 1:1 molar relationship in an enteric coated form. It is used in the UK, Canada, and U.S. for the treatment of the manic episodes of bipolar disorder. In rare cases, it is also used as a treatment for major depressive disorder, and increasingly taken long-term for prevention of both manic and depressive phases of bipolar disorder, especially the rapid-cycling variant.
Phosphodiesterase	A Phosphodiesterase is any enzyme that breaks a phosphodiester bond. Usually, people speaking of Phosphodiesterase are referring to cyclic nucleotide Phosphodiesterases, which have great clinical significance and are described below. However, many other enzyme families are, in the technical sense, Phosphodiesterases, including phospholipases C and D, autotaxin, sphingomyelin Phosphodiesterase, DNases, RNases, and restriction endonucleases (which all break the phosphodiester backbone of DNA or RNA), as well as numerous less-well-characterized small-molecule Phosphodiesterases.

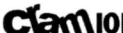

Chapter 5. Ion Channels and Enzymes Targets of Psychopharmacological Drug Action

Phosphorylation	Phosphorylation is the addition of a phosphate (PO_4^{3-}) group to a protein or other organic molecule. Phosphorylation activates or deactivates many protein enzymes. Protein phosphorylation in particular plays a significant role in a wide range of cellular processes.
Anticonvulsant	The anticonvulsants are a diverse group of pharmaceuticals used in the treatment of epileptic seizures. anticonvulsants are also increasingly being used in the treatment of bipolar disorder, since many seem to act as mood stabilizers. The goal of an anticonvulsant is to suppress the rapid and excessive firing of neurons that start a seizure.
Chronic pain	Chronic pain has several different meanings in medicine. Traditionally, the distinction between acute and chronic pain has relied upon an arbitrary interval of time from onset; the two most commonly used markers being 3 months and 6 months since the initiation of pain, though some theorists and researchers have placed the transition from acute to chronic pain at 12 months. Others apply acute to pain that lasts less than 30 days, chronic to pain of more than six months duration, and subacute to pain that lasts from one to six months.
Huntington's disease	Huntington's disease is a neurodegenerative genetic disorder that affects muscle coordination and leads to cognitive decline and dementia. It typically becomes noticeable in middle age. Huntington's disease is the most common genetic cause of abnormal involuntary writhing movements called chorea.
Mania	Mania is a state of abnormally elevated or irritable mood, arousal, and/ or energy levels, which is a criterion for certain psychiatric diagnoses; usually, it is a form of clinical psychosis. There are several possible causes f outside of mood disorders, including drug abuse and brain tumors, but it is most often associated with bipolar disorder, where episodes of Mania alternate with episodes of major depression. These cycles may relate to diurnal rhythms and environmental stressors.
Narcolepsy	Narcolepsy is a chronic sleep disorder, or dyssomnia. The condition is characterized by excessive daytime sleepiness (EDS) in which a person experiences extreme fatigue and possibly falls asleep at inappropriate times, such as while at work or at school. A narcoleptic will most likely experience disturbed nocturnal sleep and also abnormal daytime sleep pattern, which is often confused with insomnia.

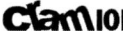

Chapter 5. Ion Channels and Enzymes Targets of Psychopharmacological Drug Action

Channel blocker	A channel blocker is a type of drug which binds inside the pore of a specific type of ion channel and blocks the flow of ions through it, resulting in an alteration of the electrochemical gradient of the cell membrane of neurons and therefore a change in neurotransmission.
Neurotransmitters	Neurotransmitters are endogenous chemicals which relay, amplify, and modulate signals between a neuron and another cell. Neurotransmitters are packaged into synaptic vesicles that cluster beneath the membrane on the presynaptic side of a synapse, and are released into the synaptic cleft, where they bind to receptors in the membrane on the postsynaptic side of the synapse. Release of Neurotransmitters usually follows arrival of an action potential at the synapse, but may follow graded electrical potentials.
Folinic acid	Folinic acid or leucovorin (USAN), generally administered as calcium or sodium folinate (or leucovorin calcium/sodium), is an adjuvant used in cancer chemotherapy involving the drug methotrexate. It is also used in synergistic combination with the chemotherapy agent 5-fluorouracil. LevoFolinic acid and its salts are the enantiopure drugs.
Psychopharmacology	Psychopharmacology is the study of drug-induced changes in mood, sensation, thinking, and behavior. The field of Psychopharmacology studies a wide range of substances with various types of psychoactive properties. The professional and commercial fields of pharmacology and Psychopharmacology do not mainly focus on psychedelic or recreational drugs, as the majority of studies are conducted for the development, study, and use of drugs for the modification of behavior and the alleviation of symptoms, particularly in the treatment of mental disorders .
Gabapentin	Gabapentin is a GABA analogue. It was originally developed for the treatment of epilepsy, and currently, Gabapentin is widely used to relieve pain, especially neuropathic pain. Gabapentin was initially synthesized to mimic the chemical structure of the neurotransmitter gamma-aminobutyric acid (GABA), but is not believed to act on the same brain receptors.
Levetiracetam	Levetiracetam (INN) is an anticonvulsant medication used to treat epilepsy. It is S-enantiomer of etiracetam, structurally similar to the prototypical nootropic drug piracetam. Levetiracetam is marketed under the trade name Keppra.

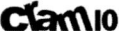

Chapter 5. Ion Channels and Enzymes Targets of Psychopharmacological Drug Action

Ligand	In coordination chemistry, a ligand is an ion or molecule that binds to a central metal atom to form a coordination complex. The bonding between metal and ligand generally involves formal donation of one or more of the ligand's electron pairs. The nature of metal-ligand bonding can range from covalent to ionic.
Pregabalin	Pregabalin is an anticonvulsant drug used for neuropathic pain and as an adjunct therapy for partial seizures with or without secondary generalization in adults. It has also been found effective for generalized anxiety disorder and is approved for this use in the European Union. It was designed as a more potent successor to gabapentin.
Mood stabilizer	A Mood stabilizer is a psychiatric medication used to treat mood disorders characterized by intense and sustained mood shifts, which is not the same as 'feeling good one minute and then bad the next.' One use is in bipolar disorder, where Mood stabilizers suppress swings between mania and depression. These drugs are also used in borderline personality disorder. Most Mood stabilizers are purely antimanic agents, meaning that they are effective at treating mania and mood cycling and shifting, but are not effective at treating depression.
Abuse	Abuse is defined as:
Cocaine	Cocaine is a crystalline tropane alkaloid that is obtained from the leaves of the coca plant. The name comes from 'coca' in addition to the alkaloid suffix -ine, forming Cocaine. It is a stimulant of the central nervous system and an appetite suppressant.
Enzyme	Enzymes are proteins that catalyze (i.e., increase the rates of) chemical reactions. In enzymatic reactions, the molecules at the beginning of the process are called substrates, and the Enzyme converts them into different molecules, called the products. Almost all processes in a biological cell need Enzymes to occur at significant rates.
Enzyme inhibitors	Enzyme inhibitors are molecules that bind to enzymes and decrease their activity. Since blocking an enzyme's activity can kill a pathogen or correct a metabolic imbalance, many drugs are Enzyme inhibitors. They are also used as herbicides and pesticides.

Chapter 5. Ion Channels and Enzymes Targets of Psychopharmacological Drug Action

Acetylcholinesterase	Acetylcholinesterase is an enzyme that degrades (through its hydrolytic activity) the neurotransmitter acetylcholine, producing choline and an acetate group. It is mainly found at neuromuscular junctions and cholinergic nervous system, where its activity serves to terminate synaptic transmission. Acetylcholinesterase has a very high catalytic activity -- each molecule of Acetylcholinesterase degrades about 25000 molecules of acetylcholine per second.
Monoamine oxidase	L-Monoamine oxidases (MAO) (EC 1.4.3.4) are a family of enzymes that catalyze the oxidation of monoamines. They are found bound to the outer membrane of mitochondria in most cell types in the body. The enzyme was originally discovered by Mary Bernheim (née Hare) in the liver and was named tyramine oxidase.
Fibromyalgia	Fibromyalgia is also referred to as FM or FMS. Fibromyalgia is characterized by chronic widespread pain and allodynia, a heightened and painful response to pressure.
Glucocorticoid	Glucocorticoids (GC) are a class of steroid hormones that bind to the Glucocorticoid receptor (GR), which is present in almost every vertebrate animal cell. The name Glucocorticoid derives from their role in the regulation of the metabolism of glucose, their synthesis in the adrenal cortex, and their steroidal structure . GCs are part of the feedback mechanism in the immune system that turns immune activity (inflammation) down.
Hormone	A hormone is a chemical released by one or more cells that affects cells in other parts of the organism. Only a small amount of hormone is required to alter cell metabolism. It is essentially a chemical messenger that transports a signal from one cell to another.
Tyrosine	Tyrosine or 4-hydroxyphenylalanine, is one of the 20 amino acids that are used by cells to synthesize proteins. It is a non-essential amino acid with a polar side group. The word 'Tyrosine' is from the Greek tyros, meaning cheese, as it was first discovered in 1846 by German chemist Justus von Liebig in the protein casein from cheese.
Cortisol	Cortisol is a corticosteroid hormone or glucocorticoid produced by the adrenal cortex, that is part of the adrenal gland (in the zona fasciculata and the zona reticularis of the adrenal cortex). It is usually referred to as the 'stress hormone' as it is involved in response to stress and anxiety, controlled by CRH. It increases blood pressure and blood sugar, and reduces immune responses. Various synthetic forms of Cortisol are used to treat a variety of different illnesses.

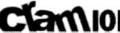

Chapter 5. Ion Channels and Enzymes Targets of Psychopharmacological Drug Action

Lithium	Lithium is a soft, silver-white metal that belongs to the alkali metal group of chemical elements. It is represented by the symbol Li, and it has the atomic number three. Under standard conditions it is the lightest metal and the least dense solid element.
MAOIs	Monoamine oxidase inhibitors (MAOIs) are a class of powerful antidepressant drugs prescribed for the treatment of depression. They are particularly effective in treating atypical depression, and have also shown efficacy in smoking cessation.
	Due to potentially lethal dietary and drug interactions, MAOIs had been reserved as a last line of defense, used only when other classes of antidepressant drugs (for example selective serotonin reuptake inhibitors and tricyclic antidepressants) have failed.
Cytokine	Cytokines are small cell-signaling protein molecules that are secreted by the glial cells of the nervous system and by numerous cells of the immune system and are a category of signaling molecules used extensively in intercellular communication. Cytokines can be classified as proteins, peptides, or glycoproteins; the term 'cytokine' encompasses a large and diverse family of regulators produced throughout the body by cells of diverse embryological origin.
Fibroblast	A fibroblast is a type of cell that synthesizes the extracellular matrix and collagen, the structural framework (stroma) for animal tissues, and plays a critical role in wound healing. Fibroblasts are the most common cells of connective tissue in animals.
Fibroblast growth factor	Fibroblast growth factors are a family of growth factors involved in angiogenesis, wound healing, and embryonic development. The Fibroblast growth factors are heparin-binding proteins and interactions with cell-surface associated heparan sulfate proteoglycans have been shown to be essential for Fibroblast growth factor signal transduction. Fibroblast growth factors are key players in the processes of proliferation and differentiation of wide variety of cells and tissues.
Hypertension	Hypertension is a chronic medical condition in which the blood pressure is elevated. It is also referred to as high blood pressure or shortened to HT, HTN or HPN. The word 'Hypertension', by itself, normally refers to systemic, arterial Hypertension.
	Hypertension can be classified as either essential (primary) or secondary.

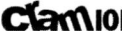

Chapter 5. Ion Channels and Enzymes Targets of Psychopharmacological Drug Action

Insulin	insulin is a hormone that has extensive effects on metabolism and other body functions, such as vascular compliance. insulin causes cells in the liver, muscle, and fat tissue to take up glucose from the blood, storing it as glycogen in the liver and muscle, and stopping use of fat as an energy source. When insulin is absent (or low), glucose is not taken up by body cells, and the body begins to use fat as an energy source, for example, by transfer of lipids from adipose tissue to the liver for mobilization as an energy source.
Interferons	interferons are proteins made and released by the cells of most vertebrates in response to the presence of pathogens -- such as viruses, bacteria, or parasites -- or tumor cells. They allow communication between cells to trigger the protective defenses of the immune system that eradicate pathogens or tumors. IFNs belong to the large class of glycoproteins known as cytokines.
Interleukins	Interleukins are a group of cytokines (secreted proteins/signaling molecules) that were first seen to be expressed by white blood cells (leukocytes). The term interleukin derives from (inter-) 'as a means of communication', and (-leukin) 'deriving from the fact that many of these proteins are produced by leukocytes and act on leukocytes'. The name is something of a relic though (the term was coined by Dr. Paetkau, University of Victoria); it has since been found that Interleukins are produced by a wide variety of body cells.
Leptin	Leptin is a 16 kDa protein hormone that plays a key role in regulating energy intake and energy expenditure, including appetite and metabolism. It is one of the most important adipose derived hormones. The Ob gene (Ob for obese, Lep for Leptin) is located on chromosome 7 in humans.
Necrosis	Necrosis is the premature death of cells and living tissue. Necrosis is caused by external factors, such as infection, toxins or trauma. This is in contrast to apoptosis, which is a naturally occurring cause of cellular death.
Tumor	A tumor or tumour is the name for a swelling or lesion formed by an abnormal growth of cells (termed neoplastic). tumor is not synonymous with cancer. A tumor can be benign, pre-malignant or malignant, whereas cancer is by definition malignant.

Chapter 6. Psychiatric Genetics

Psychiatry	Psychiatry is the medical specialty devoted to the study and treatment of mental disorders. These mental disorders include various affective, behavioural, cognitive and perceptual abnormalities. The term was first coined by the German physician Johann Christian Reil in 1808, and literally means the 'medical treatment of the mind' .
Receptor	In biochemistry, a receptor is a protein molecule, embedded in either the plasma membrane or the cytoplasm of a cell, to which one or more specific kinds of signaling molecules may attach. A molecule which binds (attaches) to a receptor is called a ligand, and may be a peptide (short protein) or other small molecule, such as a neurotransmitter, a hormone, a pharmaceutical drug, or a toxin. Each kind of receptor can bind only certain ligand shapes.
Huntington's disease	Huntington's disease is a neurodegenerative genetic disorder that affects muscle coordination and leads to cognitive decline and dementia. It typically becomes noticeable in middle age. Huntington's disease is the most common genetic cause of abnormal involuntary writhing movements called chorea.
Mental disorder	A mental disorder is a psychological or behavioral pattern generally associated with subjective distress or disability that occurs in an individual, and which is not a part of normal development or culture. Such a disorder may consist of a combination of affective, behavioural, cognitive and perceptual components. The recognition and understanding of mental health conditions have changed over time and across cultures, and there are still variations in the definition, assessment, and classification of mental disorders, although standard guideline criteria are widely accepted.
Rheumatology	Rheumatology is a sub-specialty in internal medicine and pediatrics, devoted to diagnosis and therapy of conditions and diseases affecting joints, muscles, and bones. Clinicians who specialize in rheumatology are called rheumatologists. Rheumatologists deal mainly with clinical problems involving joints, soft tissues, certain autoimmune diseases, vasculitis, and heritable connective tissue disorders.
Fibromyalgia	Fibromyalgia is also referred to as FM or FMS. Fibromyalgia is characterized by chronic widespread pain and allodynia, a heightened and painful response to pressure.
Syndrome	In medicine and psychology, a Syndrome is the association of several clinically recognizable features, signs (observed by a physician), symptoms (reported by the patient), phenomena or characteristics that often occur together, so that the presence of one feature alerts the physician to the presence of the others. In recent decades, the term has been used outside medicine to refer to a combination of phenomena seen in association.

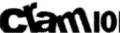

Chapter 6. Psychiatric Genetics

	The term Syndrome derives from its Greek roots and means literally 'run together', as the features do.
Prolixin	Fluphenazine is a typical antipsychotic drug used for the treatment of psychoses such as schizophrenia and acute manic phases of bipolar disorder. It belongs to the piperazine class of phenothiazines and is extremely potent; more potent than haloperidol and around fifty to seventy times the potency of chlorpromazine. It is marketed under the brand name of Prolixin and Sydocate(Surge Laboratories).
Hypertension	Hypertension is a chronic medical condition in which the blood pressure is elevated. It is also referred to as high blood pressure or shortened to HT, HTN or HPN. The word 'Hypertension', by itself, normally refers to systemic, arterial Hypertension. Hypertension can be classified as either essential (primary) or secondary.
Benadryl	Benadryl is a brand name allergy medicine marketed over-the-counter by Johnson ' Johnson subsidiary McNeil Consumer Healthcare. Prior to 2007, Benadryl was marketed by Pfizer Consumer Healthcare. Benadryl is used as an antihistamine for the temporary relief of seasonal and perennial allergy symptoms.
Phenotype	A Phenotype is any observable characteristic or trait of an organism: such as its morphology, development, biochemical or physiological properties, or behavior. Phenotypes result from the expression of an organism's genes as well as the influence of environmental factors and possible interactions between the two. The genotype of an organism is the inherited instructions it carries within its genetic code.
Resonance	In physics, resonance is the tendency of a system to oscillate with larger amplitude at some frequencies than at others. These are known as the system's resonant frequencies. At these frequencies, even small periodic driving forces can produce large amplitude oscillations, because the system stores vibrational energy.
Abuse	Abuse is defined as:
Cocaine	Cocaine is a crystalline tropane alkaloid that is obtained from the leaves of the coca plant. The name comes from 'coca' in addition to the alkaloid suffix -ine, forming Cocaine. It is a stimulant of the central nervous system and an appetite suppressant.

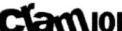

Chapter 6. Psychiatric Genetics

Schizophrenia	Schizophrenia , from the Greek roots skhizein and phrÄ"n, phren- (φρÎ®ν, φρεν-; 'mind') is a psychiatric diagnosis that describes a neuropsychiatric and mental disorder characterized by abnormalities in the perception or expression of reality. It most commonly manifests as auditory hallucinations, paranoid or bizarre delusions, or disorganized speech and thinking with significant social or occupational dysfunction. Onset of symptoms typically occurs in young adulthood, with around 0.4-0.6% of the population affected.
Insomnia	Insomnia is a symptom which can accompany several sleep, medical and psychiatric disorders, characterized by persistent difficulty falling asleep and/or staying asleep despite the opportunity. Insomnia is typically followed by functional impairment while awake. Both organic and non-organic Insomnia without other cause constitute a sleep disorder, primary Insomnia.
Huntington's disease	Huntington's disease is a neurodegenerative genetic disorder that affects muscle coordination and leads to cognitive decline and dementia. It typically becomes noticeable in middle age. Huntington's disease is the most common genetic cause of abnormal involuntary writhing movements called chorea.
Narcolepsy	Narcolepsy is a chronic sleep disorder, or dyssomnia. The condition is characterized by excessive daytime sleepiness (EDS) in which a person experiences extreme fatigue and possibly falls asleep at inappropriate times, such as while at work or at school. A narcoleptic will most likely experience disturbed nocturnal sleep and also abnormal daytime sleep pattern, which is often confused with insomnia.

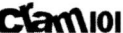

Chapter 7. Circuits in Psychopharmacology

Symptom	A Symptom is a departure from normal function or feeling which is noticed by a patient, indicating the presence of disease or abnormality. A Symptom is subjective, observed by the patient, and not measured.
Receptor	In biochemistry, a receptor is a protein molecule, embedded in either the plasma membrane or the cytoplasm of a cell, to which one or more specific kinds of signaling molecules may attach. A molecule which binds (attaches) to a receptor is called a ligand, and may be a peptide (short protein) or other small molecule, such as a neurotransmitter, a hormone, a pharmaceutical drug, or a toxin. Each kind of receptor can bind only certain ligand shapes.
Schizophrenia	Schizophrenia , from the Greek roots skhizein and phrÄ"n, phren- (φρÎ®ν, φρεν-; 'mind') is a psychiatric diagnosis that describes a neuropsychiatric and mental disorder characterized by abnormalities in the perception or expression of reality. It most commonly manifests as auditory hallucinations, paranoid or bizarre delusions, or disorganized speech and thinking with significant social or occupational dysfunction. Onset of symptoms typically occurs in young adulthood, with around 0.4-0.6% of the population affected.
Psychopharmacology	Psychopharmacology is the study of drug-induced changes in mood, sensation, thinking, and behavior. The field of Psychopharmacology studies a wide range of substances with various types of psychoactive properties. The professional and commercial fields of pharmacology and Psychopharmacology do not mainly focus on psychedelic or recreational drugs, as the majority of studies are conducted for the development, study, and use of drugs for the modification of behavior and the alleviation of symptoms, particularly in the treatment of mental disorders .
Dopaminergic	Dopaminergic means related to the neurotransmitter dopamine. For example, certain proteins such as the dopamine transporter (DAT), vesicular monoamine transporter 2 ($VMAT_2$), and dopamine receptors can be classified as Dopaminergic, and neurons which synthesize or contain dopamine and synapses with dopamine receptors in them may also be labeled as Dopaminergic. Enzymes which regulate the biosynthesis or metabolism of dopamine such as aromatic L-amino acid decarboxylase (AAAD) or DOPA decarboxylase (DDC), monoamine oxidase (MAO), and catechol O-methyl transferase (COMT) may be referred to as Dopaminergic as well.
Iloperidone	Iloperidone is an atypical antipsychotic for the treatment of schizophrenia. It was approved by the U.S. Food and Drug Administration (FDA) for use in the United States on May 6, 2009.

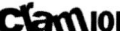

Chapter 7. Circuits in Psychopharmacology

Amitriptyline	Amitriptyline is a psychoactive drug and pharmaceutical of the tricyclic antidepressant (TCA) chemical class which is used primarily as an antidepressant and anxiolytic agent. It is the most widely prescribed TCA and perhaps also the most efficient against depressive symptoms.
	Amitriptyline is approved for the treatment of major depression.
Agonist	An Agonist is a drug that binds to a receptor of a cell and triggers a response by the cell. An Agonist often mimics the action of a naturally occurring substance.
	An Agonist produces an action.
Huntington's disease	Huntington's disease is a neurodegenerative genetic disorder that affects muscle coordination and leads to cognitive decline and dementia. It typically becomes noticeable in middle age. Huntington's disease is the most common genetic cause of abnormal involuntary writhing movements called chorea.
Dopamine	Dopamine is a neurotransmitter that occurs in a wide variety of animals, including both vertebrates and invertebrates. In the brain, this phenethylamine functions as a neurotransmitter, activating the five types of Dopamine receptors--D_1, D_2, D_3, D_4, and D_5--and their variants. Dopamine is produced in several areas of the brain, including the substantia nigra and the ventral tegmental area.
Neurotransmitters	Neurotransmitters are endogenous chemicals which relay, amplify, and modulate signals between a neuron and another cell. Neurotransmitters are packaged into synaptic vesicles that cluster beneath the membrane on the presynaptic side of a synapse, and are released into the synaptic cleft, where they bind to receptors in the membrane on the postsynaptic side of the synapse. Release of Neurotransmitters usually follows arrival of an action potential at the synapse, but may follow graded electrical potentials.
Insomnia	Insomnia is a symptom which can accompany several sleep, medical and psychiatric disorders, characterized by persistent difficulty falling asleep and/or staying asleep despite the opportunity. Insomnia is typically followed by functional impairment while awake. Both organic and non-organic Insomnia without other cause constitute a sleep disorder, primary Insomnia.

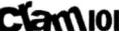

CramI0I

Chapter 7. Circuits in Psychopharmacology

Mesencephalon	In biological anatomy, the Mesencephalon comprises the tectum (or corpora quadrigemini), tegmentum, the ventricular mesocoelia (or 'iter'), and the cerebral peduncles, as well as several nuclei and fasciculi. Caudally the Mesencephalon adjoins the pons (metencephalon) and rostrally it adjoins the diencephalon (Thalamus, hypothalamus, et al). During development, the Mesencephalon forms from the middle of three vesicles that arise from the neural tube to generate the brain.
Zaleplon	Zaleplon is a sedative/hypnotic, mainly used for insomnia. It is a nonbenzodiazepine hypnotic from the pyrazolopyrimidine class. In terms of adverse effects Zaleplon appears to offer little improvement compared to both benzodiazepines and other non-benzodiazepine Z-drugs.
Ziprasidone	Ziprasidone was the fifth atypical antipsychotic to gain FDA approval (February 2001). In the United States, Ziprasidone is Food and Drug Administration (FDA) approved for the treatment of schizophrenia, and the intramuscular injection form of Ziprasidone is approved for acute agitation in schizophrenic patients. Ziprasidone has also received approval for acute treatment of mania and mixed states associated with bipolar disorder.
Norepinephrine	Noradrenaline (BAN) is a catecholamine with dual roles as a hormone and a neurotransmitter. As a stress hormone, Norepinephrine affects parts of the brain where attention and responding actions are controlled. Along with epinephrine, Norepinephrine also underlies the fight-or-flight response, directly increasing heart rate, triggering the release of glucose from energy stores, and increasing blood flow to skeletal muscle.
Quetiapine	Quetiapine fumarate , marketed by AstraZeneca as Seroquel or SeroquelXR and by Orion Pharma as Ketipinor, is an atypical antipsychotic used in the management of schizophrenia, bipolar I mania, bipolar II depression, bipolar I depression, and used off-label for a variety of other purposes, including insomnia and anxiety disorders. Annual sales are approx. $4.7bn worldwide, and $2.9bn in the US. The US patent, which was set to expire in 2011, received a pediatric exclusivity extension which pushed its expiration to March 26, 2012; however, in Canada it has already expired.

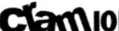

Chapter 7. Circuits in Psychopharmacology

Serotonin	Serotonin is a monoamine neurotransmitter. Biochemically derived from tryptophan, serotonin is primarily found in the gastrointestinal (GI) tract, platelets, and in the central nervous system (CNS) of animals including humans. It is a well-known contributor to feelings of well-being; therefore it is also known as a 'happiness hormone' despite not being a hormone.
Acetylcholine	The chemical compound Acetylcholine is a neurotransmitter in both the peripheral nervous system (PNS) and central nervous system (CNS) in many organisms including humans. Acetylcholine is one of many neurotransmitters in the autonomic nervous system (ANS) and the only neurotransmitter used in the motor division of the somatic nervous system. (Sensory neurons use glutamate and various peptides at their synapses).
Cholinergic	A receptor is cholinergic if it uses acetylcholine as its neurotransmitter. cholinergic means related to the neurotransmitter acetylcholine, and is typically used in a neurological perspective. The parasympathetic nervous system is entirely cholinergic.
Atrophy	Atrophy is the partial or complete wasting away of a part of the body. Causes of Atrophy include poor nourishment, poor circulation, loss of hormonal support, loss of nerve supply to the target organ, disuse or lack of exercise or disease intrinsic to the tissue itself. Hormonal and nerve inputs that maintain an organ or body part are referred to as trophic [noun] in medical practice.
Glucocorticoid	Glucocorticoids (GC) are a class of steroid hormones that bind to the Glucocorticoid receptor (GR), which is present in almost every vertebrate animal cell. The name Glucocorticoid derives from their role in the regulation of the metabolism of glucose, their synthesis in the adrenal cortex, and their steroidal structure . GCs are part of the feedback mechanism in the immune system that turns immune activity (inflammation) down.
Interaction	Interaction is a kind of action that occurs as two or more objects have an effect upon one another. The idea of a two-way effect is essential in the concept of Interaction, as opposed to a one-way causal effect. A closely related term is interconnectivity, which deals with the Interactions of Interactions within systems: combinations of many simple Interactions can lead to surprising emergent phenomena.

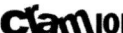

Chapter 7. Circuits in Psychopharmacology

Tolerance	Toleration and Tolerance are terms used in social, cultural and religious contexts to describe attitudes which are 'tolerant' (or moderately respectful) of practices or group memberships that may be disapproved of by those in the majority. In practice, 'Tolerance' indicates support for practices that prohibit ethnic and religious discrimination. Conversely, 'inTolerance' may be used to refer to the discriminatory practices sought to be prohibited.
Anxiety disorder	Anxiety disorder is a blanket term covering several different forms of abnormal and pathological fear and anxiety which only came under the aegis of psychiatry at the very end of the 19th century. Current psychiatric diagnostic criteria recognize a wide variety of Anxiety disorders. Recent surveys have found that as many as 18% of Americans may be affected by one or more of them.
Abuse	Abuse is defined as:
Cocaine	Cocaine is a crystalline tropane alkaloid that is obtained from the leaves of the coca plant. The name comes from 'coca' in addition to the alkaloid suffix -ine, forming Cocaine. It is a stimulant of the central nervous system and an appetite suppressant.
Estrogen	Estrogens (U.S., otherwise oEstrogens or Ästrogens) are a group of steroid compounds and functioning as the primary female sex hormone, their name comes from estrus/oistros (period of fertility for female mammals) + gen/gonos = to generate.
	Estrogens are used as part of some oral contraceptives, in Estrogen replacement therapy for postmenopausal women, and in hormone replacement therapy for trans women.
	Like all steroid hormones, Estrogens readily diffuse across the cell membrane.
Deficiency	A Deficiency is a lack of something. Example
	there is a Deficiency of oxygen in the air and we shall soon suffocate.
	· In mathematics, a deficient number is a number n for which $\sigma(n) < 2n$.
	· In medicine there are a variety of nutrient deficiencies:
	· Avitaminosis is a Deficiency of vitamins.
	· Boron Deficiency

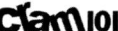

Chapter 7. Circuits in Psychopharmacology

	· Chromium Deficiency
	· Iron Deficiency
	· Iodine Deficiency
	· Magnesium Deficiency
	· Micronutrient Deficiency
	· In construction, a Deficiency is an item, or condition that is considered sub-standard, or below minimum expectations, such as those mandated by either drawings or specifications or the building code or the fire code, and/or any combination of the foregoing. Deficiencies are routinely discussed and dealt with in construction site meetings.
	· In genetics, a genetic deletion is also called a Deficiency.
	· In real estate law, a Deficiency in the ability to pay off a debt is called a Deficiency judgment or Deficiency judgement.
Folate deficiency	Folate deficiency is a lack of folic acid in the diet and the signs are often subtle.
	Loss of appetite, and weight loss can occur. Additional signs are weakness, sore tongue, headaches, heart palpitations, irritability, and behavioral disorders.

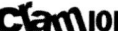

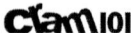

Chapter 8. From Circuits to Symptoms in Psychopharmacology

Iloperidone	Iloperidone is an atypical antipsychotic for the treatment of schizophrenia. It was approved by the U.S. Food and Drug Administration (FDA) for use in the United States on May 6, 2009.
Neurotransmitters	Neurotransmitters are endogenous chemicals which relay, amplify, and modulate signals between a neuron and another cell. Neurotransmitters are packaged into synaptic vesicles that cluster beneath the membrane on the presynaptic side of a synapse, and are released into the synaptic cleft, where they bind to receptors in the membrane on the postsynaptic side of the synapse. Release of Neurotransmitters usually follows arrival of an action potential at the synapse, but may follow graded electrical potentials.
Symptom	A Symptom is a departure from normal function or feeling which is noticed by a patient, indicating the presence of disease or abnormality. A Symptom is subjective, observed by the patient, and not measured.
Trauma	Trauma can represent:

Trauma can represent:

· Physical Trauma, an often serious and body-altering physical injury, such as the removal of a limb

· Blunt Trauma, a type of physical Trauma caused by impact or other force applied from or with a blunt object

· Penetrating Trauma, a type of physical Trauma in which the skin or tissues are pierced by an object

· Psychological Trauma, an emotional or psychological injury, usually resulting from an extremely stressful or life-threatening situation

· Post-cult Trauma, the intense emotional problems that some members of cults and new religious movements experience upon disaffection and disaffiliation

· Trauma team, a group of healthcare workers who attend to seriously ill or injured casualties who arrive at a hospital emergency department

· Trauma center, a hospital equipped to provide comprehensive emergency medical services to patients suffering Traumatic injuries

· Trauma, a character associated with Avengers: The Initiative in the Marvel Universe

· Trauma an American film directed by Robert M. Young

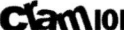

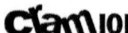

Chapter 8. From Circuits to Symptoms in Psychopharmacology

	· Trauma a horror film directed by Dario Argento
	· Trauma a psychological thriller directed by Marc Evans and starring Colin Firth
	· Trauma a medical drama set in San Francisco
	· Also see Troma Entertainment, a film company specializing in independent, horror, and exploitation films
	· Trauma Studios, an American computer game development company
	· Trauma Center (series), a surgical based video game.
	· 'Day Twelve: Trauma', a song by Ayreon on the album The Human Equation
	· 'Trauma' (song) by Ayumi Hamasaki
	· Trauma by rapper/producer DJ Quik
	· Trauma Records, a record label
	· Trauma Flintstone, drag performer and actress
	· Baltimore Trauma, professional paintball team from North Carolina
Benadryl	Benadryl is a brand name allergy medicine marketed over-the-counter by Johnson ' Johnson subsidiary McNeil Consumer Healthcare. Prior to 2007, Benadryl was marketed by Pfizer Consumer Healthcare. Benadryl is used as an antihistamine for the temporary relief of seasonal and perennial allergy symptoms.
Atrophy	Atrophy is the partial or complete wasting away of a part of the body. Causes of Atrophy include poor nourishment, poor circulation, loss of hormonal support, loss of nerve supply to the target organ, disuse or lack of exercise or disease intrinsic to the tissue itself. Hormonal and nerve inputs that maintain an organ or body part are referred to as trophic [noun] in medical practice.
Huntington's disease	Huntington's disease is a neurodegenerative genetic disorder that affects muscle coordination and leads to cognitive decline and dementia. It typically becomes noticeable in middle age. Huntington's disease is the most common genetic cause of abnormal involuntary writhing movements called chorea.

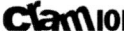

Chapter 8. From Circuits to Symptoms in Psychopharmacology

Huntington's disease	Huntington's disease is a neurodegenerative genetic disorder that affects muscle coordination and leads to cognitive decline and dementia. It typically becomes noticeable in middle age. Huntington's disease is the most common genetic cause of abnormal involuntary writhing movements called chorea.
Receptor	In biochemistry, a receptor is a protein molecule, embedded in either the plasma membrane or the cytoplasm of a cell, to which one or more specific kinds of signaling molecules may attach. A molecule which binds (attaches) to a receptor is called a ligand, and may be a peptide (short protein) or other small molecule, such as a neurotransmitter, a hormone, a pharmaceutical drug, or a toxin. Each kind of receptor can bind only certain ligand shapes.
Syndrome	In medicine and psychology, a Syndrome is the association of several clinically recognizable features, signs (observed by a physician), symptoms (reported by the patient), phenomena or characteristics that often occur together, so that the presence of one feature alerts the physician to the presence of the others. In recent decades, the term has been used outside medicine to refer to a combination of phenomena seen in association. The term Syndrome derives from its Greek roots and means literally 'run together', as the features do.
Insomnia	Insomnia is a symptom which can accompany several sleep, medical and psychiatric disorders, characterized by persistent difficulty falling asleep and/or staying asleep despite the opportunity. Insomnia is typically followed by functional impairment while awake. Both organic and non-organic Insomnia without other cause constitute a sleep disorder, primary Insomnia.
Resonance	In physics, resonance is the tendency of a system to oscillate with larger amplitude at some frequencies than at others. These are known as the system's resonant frequencies. At these frequencies, even small periodic driving forces can produce large amplitude oscillations, because the system stores vibrational energy.
Serotonin	Serotonin is a monoamine neurotransmitter. Biochemically derived from tryptophan, serotonin is primarily found in the gastrointestinal (GI) tract, platelets, and in the central nervous system (CNS) of animals including humans. It is a well-known contributor to feelings of well-being; therefore it is also known as a 'happiness hormone' despite not being a hormone.

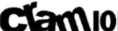

Chapter 8. From Circuits to Symptoms in Psychopharmacology

Dopamine	Dopamine is a neurotransmitter that occurs in a wide variety of animals, including both vertebrates and invertebrates. In the brain, this phenethylamine functions as a neurotransmitter, activating the five types of Dopamine receptors--D_1, D_2, D_3, D_4, and D_5--and their variants. Dopamine is produced in several areas of the brain, including the substantia nigra and the ventral tegmental area.
Phosphatase	A Phosphatase is an enzyme that removes a phosphate group from its substrate by hydrolysing phosphoric acid monoesters into a phosphate ion and a molecule with a free hydroxyl group . This action is directly opposite to that of phosphorylases and kinases, which attach phosphate groups to their substrates by using energetic molecules like ATP. A common Phosphatase in many organisms is alkaline Phosphatase. Protein phosphorylation is the most common and important form of reversible protein posttranslational modification (PTM), with up to 30% of all proteins being phosphorylated at any given time.
Psychopharmacology	Psychopharmacology is the study of drug-induced changes in mood, sensation, thinking, and behavior. The field of Psychopharmacology studies a wide range of substances with various types of psychoactive properties. The professional and commercial fields of pharmacology and Psychopharmacology do not mainly focus on psychedelic or recreational drugs, as the majority of studies are conducted for the development, study, and use of drugs for the modification of behavior and the alleviation of symptoms, particularly in the treatment of mental disorders .
Deficiency	A Deficiency is a lack of something. Example there is a Deficiency of oxygen in the air and we shall soon suffocate. · In mathematics, a deficient number is a number n for which $\sigma(n) < 2n$. · In medicine there are a variety of nutrient deficiencies: · Avitaminosis is a Deficiency of vitamins. · Boron Deficiency · Chromium Deficiency · Iron Deficiency

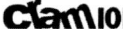

· Iodine Deficiency

· Magnesium Deficiency

· Micronutrient Deficiency

· In construction, a Deficiency is an item, or condition that is considered sub-standard, or below minimum expectations, such as those mandated by either drawings or specifications or the building code or the fire code, and/or any combination of the foregoing. Deficiencies are routinely discussed and dealt with in construction site meetings.

· In genetics, a genetic deletion is also called a Deficiency.

· In real estate law, a Deficiency in the ability to pay off a debt is called a Deficiency judgment or Deficiency judgement.

Anxiety disorder	Anxiety disorder is a blanket term covering several different forms of abnormal and pathological fear and anxiety which only came under the aegis of psychiatry at the very end of the 19th century. Current psychiatric diagnostic criteria recognize a wide variety of Anxiety disorders. Recent surveys have found that as many as 18% of Americans may be affected by one or more of them.
Schizophrenia	Schizophrenia , from the Greek roots skhizein and phrÄ"n, phren- (φρÎ®ν, φρεν-; 'mind') is a psychiatric diagnosis that describes a neuropsychiatric and mental disorder characterized by abnormalities in the perception or expression of reality. It most commonly manifests as auditory hallucinations, paranoid or bizarre delusions, or disorganized speech and thinking with significant social or occupational dysfunction. Onset of symptoms typically occurs in young adulthood, with around 0.4-0.6% of the population affected.
Acetylcholine	The chemical compound Acetylcholine is a neurotransmitter in both the peripheral nervous system (PNS) and central nervous system (CNS) in many organisms including humans. Acetylcholine is one of many neurotransmitters in the autonomic nervous system (ANS) and the only neurotransmitter used in the motor division of the somatic nervous system. (Sensory neurons use glutamate and various peptides at their synapses).

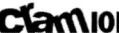

Chapter 8. From Circuits to Symptoms in Psychopharmacology

Glucocorticoid	Glucocorticoids (GC) are a class of steroid hormones that bind to the Glucocorticoid receptor (GR), which is present in almost every vertebrate animal cell. The name Glucocorticoid derives from their role in the regulation of the metabolism of glucose, their synthesis in the adrenal cortex, and their steroidal structure .
	GCs are part of the feedback mechanism in the immune system that turns immune activity (inflammation) down.
Histamine	Histamine is a biogenic amine involved in local immune responses as well as regulating physiological function in the gut and acting as a neurotransmitter. Histamine triggers the inflammatory response. As part of an immune response to foreign pathogens, Histamine is produced by basophils and by mast cells found in nearby connective tissues.
Quetiapine	Quetiapine fumarate , marketed by AstraZeneca as Seroquel or SeroquelXR and by Orion Pharma as Ketipinor, is an atypical antipsychotic used in the management of schizophrenia, bipolar I mania, bipolar II depression, bipolar I depression, and used off-label for a variety of other purposes, including insomnia and anxiety disorders.
	Annual sales are approx. $4.7bn worldwide, and $2.9bn in the US. The US patent, which was set to expire in 2011, received a pediatric exclusivity extension which pushed its expiration to March 26, 2012; however, in Canada it has already expired.

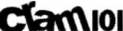

Chapter 9. Psychosis and Schizophrenia

Psychosis	Psychosis means abnormal condition of the mind, and is a generic psychiatric term for a mental state often described as involving a 'loss of contact with reality'. People suffering from Psychosis are said to be psychotic.
	People experiencing Psychosis may report hallucinations or delusional beliefs, and may exhibit personality changes and thought disorder.
Haloperidol	Haloperidol is a typical antipsychotic. It is in the butyrophenone class of antipsychotic medications and has pharmacological effects similar to the phenothiazines.
	Haloperidol is an older antipsychotic used in the treatment of schizophrenia and, more acutely, in the treatment of acute psychotic states and delirium.
Huntington's disease	Huntington's disease is a neurodegenerative genetic disorder that affects muscle coordination and leads to cognitive decline and dementia. It typically becomes noticeable in middle age. Huntington's disease is the most common genetic cause of abnormal involuntary writhing movements called chorea.
Receptor	In biochemistry, a receptor is a protein molecule, embedded in either the plasma membrane or the cytoplasm of a cell, to which one or more specific kinds of signaling molecules may attach. A molecule which binds (attaches) to a receptor is called a ligand, and may be a peptide (short protein) or other small molecule, such as a neurotransmitter, a hormone, a pharmaceutical drug, or a toxin. Each kind of receptor can bind only certain ligand shapes.
Symptom	A Symptom is a departure from normal function or feeling which is noticed by a patient, indicating the presence of disease or abnormality. A Symptom is subjective, observed by the patient, and not measured.
Syndrome	In medicine and psychology, a Syndrome is the association of several clinically recognizable features, signs (observed by a physician), symptoms (reported by the patient), phenomena or characteristics that often occur together, so that the presence of one feature alerts the physician to the presence of the others. In recent decades, the term has been used outside medicine to refer to a combination of phenomena seen in association.
	The term Syndrome derives from its Greek roots and means literally 'run together', as the features do.

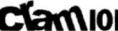

Chapter 9. Psychosis and Schizophrenia

Agonist	An Agonist is a drug that binds to a receptor of a cell and triggers a response by the cell. An Agonist often mimics the action of a naturally occurring substance. An Agonist produces an action.
Antihistamine	A histamine antagonist is an agent that serves to inhibit the release or action of histamine. antihistamine can be used to describe any histamine antagonist, but it is usually reserved for the classical antihistamines that act upon the H_1 histamine receptor. antihistamines are used as treatment for allergies.
Huntington's disease	Huntington's disease is a neurodegenerative genetic disorder that affects muscle coordination and leads to cognitive decline and dementia. It typically becomes noticeable in middle age. Huntington's disease is the most common genetic cause of abnormal involuntary writhing movements called chorea.
Dopamine	Dopamine is a neurotransmitter that occurs in a wide variety of animals, including both vertebrates and invertebrates. In the brain, this phenethylamine functions as a neurotransmitter, activating the five types of Dopamine receptors--D_1, D_2, D_3, D_4, and D_5--and their variants. Dopamine is produced in several areas of the brain, including the substantia nigra and the ventral tegmental area.
Histidine	Histidine Histidine an essential amino acid, has a positively charged imidazole functional group. It is the one of the 22 proteinogenic amino acids. Its codons are CAU and CAC. Histidine was first isolated by German physician Albrecht Kossel in 1896. Histidine is an essential amino acid in humans and other mammals.
Schizophrenia	Schizophrenia , from the Greek roots skhizein and phrÄ"n, phren- (φρÎ®ν, φρεν-; 'mind') is a psychiatric diagnosis that describes a neuropsychiatric and mental disorder characterized by abnormalities in the perception or expression of reality. It most commonly manifests as auditory hallucinations, paranoid or bizarre delusions, or disorganized speech and thinking with significant social or occupational dysfunction. Onset of symptoms typically occurs in young adulthood, with around 0.4-0.6% of the population affected.
Lewy bodies	Lewy bodies are abnormal aggregates of protein that develop inside nerve cells in Parkinson's disease (PD) and some other disorders. They are identified under the microscope when histology is performed on the brain.

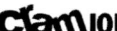

Chapter 9. Psychosis and Schizophrenia

	Lewy bodies appear as spherical masses that displace other cell components.
Cholinergic	A receptor is cholinergic if it uses acetylcholine as its neurotransmitter. cholinergic means related to the neurotransmitter acetylcholine, and is typically used in a neurological perspective. The parasympathetic nervous system is entirely cholinergic.
Aventyl	Nortriptyline is a second-generation tricyclic antidepressant marketed as the hydrochloride under the trade names Sensoval, Aventyl, Pamelor, Norpress, Allegron and Nortrilen. It is used in the treatment of major depression and childhood nocturnal enuresis (bedwetting). In addition, it is sometimes used for chronic illnesses such as chronic fatigue syndrome, chronic pain and migraines, and labile affect in some neurological conditions.
Norepinephrine	Noradrenaline (BAN) is a catecholamine with dual roles as a hormone and a neurotransmitter. As a stress hormone, Norepinephrine affects parts of the brain where attention and responding actions are controlled. Along with epinephrine, Norepinephrine also underlies the fight-or-flight response, directly increasing heart rate, triggering the release of glucose from energy stores, and increasing blood flow to skeletal muscle.
Psychopharmacology	Psychopharmacology is the study of drug-induced changes in mood, sensation, thinking, and behavior. The field of Psychopharmacology studies a wide range of substances with various types of psychoactive properties. The professional and commercial fields of pharmacology and Psychopharmacology do not mainly focus on psychedelic or recreational drugs, as the majority of studies are conducted for the development, study, and use of drugs for the modification of behavior and the alleviation of symptoms, particularly in the treatment of mental disorders .
Benadryl	Benadryl is a brand name allergy medicine marketed over-the-counter by Johnson ' Johnson subsidiary McNeil Consumer Healthcare. Prior to 2007, Benadryl was marketed by Pfizer Consumer Healthcare. Benadryl is used as an antihistamine for the temporary relief of seasonal and perennial allergy symptoms.
Schizoaffective disorder	Schizoaffective disorder is a psychiatric diagnosis that describes a mental disorder characterized by recurring episodes of elevated or depressed mood, or of simultaneously elevated and depressed mood, that alternate with, or occur together with, distortions in perception.

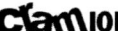

Chapter 9. Psychosis and Schizophrenia

	Schizoaffective disorder most commonly affects cognition and emotion. Auditory hallucinations, paranoia, bizarre delusions, or disorganized speech and thinking with significant social and occupational dysfunction are typical.
Rheumatology	Rheumatology is a sub-specialty in internal medicine and pediatrics, devoted to diagnosis and therapy of conditions and diseases affecting joints, muscles, and bones. Clinicians who specialize in rheumatology are called rheumatologists. Rheumatologists deal mainly with clinical problems involving joints, soft tissues, certain autoimmune diseases, vasculitis, and heritable connective tissue disorders.
Dementia	Dementia is a serious cognitive disorder. It may be static, the result of a unique global brain injury or progressive, resulting in long-term decline in cognitive function due to damage or disease in the body beyond what might be expected from normal aging. Although Dementia is far more common in the geriatric population, it may occur in any stage of adulthood.
Fibromyalgia	Fibromyalgia is also referred to as FM or FMS. Fibromyalgia is characterized by chronic widespread pain and allodynia, a heightened and painful response to pressure.
Iloperidone	Iloperidone is an atypical antipsychotic for the treatment of schizophrenia. It was approved by the U.S. Food and Drug Administration (FDA) for use in the United States on May 6, 2009.
Pharmacy	Pharmacy is the health profession that links the health sciences with the chemical sciences and it is charged with ensuring the safe and effective use of pharmaceutical drugs. The scope of pharmacy practice includes more traditional roles such as compounding and dispensing medications, and it also includes more modern services related to health care, including clinical services, reviewing medications for safety and efficacy, and providing drug information. Pharmacists, therefore, are the experts on drug therapy and are the primary health professionals who optimize medication use to provide patients with positive health outcomes.
Algorithm	In mathematics, computer science, and related subjects, an Algorithm is an effective method for solving a problem using a finite sequence of instructions. Algorithms are used for calculation, data processing, and many other fields.

	Each Algorithm is a list of well-defined instructions for completing a task.
Antidepressant	An antidepressant is a psychiatric medication used to alleviate mood disorders, such as major depression and dysthymia and anxiety disorders such as social anxiety disorder. According to Gelder, Mayou '*Geddes (2005) people with a depressive illness will experience a therapeutic effect to their mood, however this will not be experienced in healthy individuals. Drugs including the monoamine oxidase inhibitors (MAOIs), tricyclic antidepressants (TCAs), tetracyclic antidepressants (TeCAs), selective serotonin reuptake inhibitors (SSRIs), and serotonin-norepinephrine reuptake inhibitors (SNRIs) are most commonly associated with the term.
Amitriptyline	Amitriptyline is a psychoactive drug and pharmaceutical of the tricyclic antidepressant (TCA) chemical class which is used primarily as an antidepressant and anxiolytic agent. It is the most widely prescribed TCA and perhaps also the most efficient against depressive symptoms. Amitriptyline is approved for the treatment of major depression.
Dopaminergic	Dopaminergic means related to the neurotransmitter dopamine. For example, certain proteins such as the dopamine transporter (DAT), vesicular monoamine transporter 2 ($VMAT_2$), and dopamine receptors can be classified as Dopaminergic, and neurons which synthesize or contain dopamine and synapses with dopamine receptors in them may also be labeled as Dopaminergic. Enzymes which regulate the biosynthesis or metabolism of dopamine such as aromatic L-amino acid decarboxylase (AAAD) or DOPA decarboxylase (DDC), monoamine oxidase (MAO), and catechol O-methyl transferase (COMT) may be referred to as Dopaminergic as well.
Tyrosine	Tyrosine or 4-hydroxyphenylalanine, is one of the 20 amino acids that are used by cells to synthesize proteins. It is a non-essential amino acid with a polar side group. The word 'Tyrosine' is from the Greek tyros, meaning cheese, as it was first discovered in 1846 by German chemist Justus von Liebig in the protein casein from cheese.
Tyrosine hydroxylase	Tyrosine hydroxylase or tyrosine 3-monooxygenase is the enzyme responsible for catalyzing the conversion of the amino acid L-tyrosine to dihydroxyphenylalanine (DOPA). DOPA is a precursor for dopamine, which, in turn, is a precursor for norepinephrine (noradrenaline) and epinephrine (adrenaline). In humans, Tyrosine hydroxylase is encoded by the Tyrosine hydroxylase gene.
Abuse	Abuse is defined as:

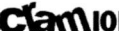

Chapter 9. Psychosis and Schizophrenia

Cocaine	Cocaine is a crystalline tropane alkaloid that is obtained from the leaves of the coca plant. The name comes from 'coca' in addition to the alkaloid suffix -ine, forming Cocaine. It is a stimulant of the central nervous system and an appetite suppressant.
Dopamine agonist	A Dopamine agonist is a compound that activates dopamine receptors in the absence of the dopamine ligand. Dopamine agonists activate signaling pathways through the dopamine receptor and trimeric G-proteins, ultimately leading to changes in gene transcription.
Acetylcholine	The chemical compound Acetylcholine is a neurotransmitter in both the peripheral nervous system (PNS) and central nervous system (CNS) in many organisms including humans. Acetylcholine is one of many neurotransmitters in the autonomic nervous system (ANS) and the only neurotransmitter used in the motor division of the somatic nervous system. (Sensory neurons use glutamate and various peptides at their synapses).
Substance abuse	Although the term substance can refer to any physical matter, Substance abuse has come to refer to the overindulgence in and dependence of a drug or other chemical leading to effects that are detrimental to the individual's physical and mental health, or the welfare of others. Source: A Public Health Approach to Drug Control in Canada, Health Officers Council of British Columbia, 2005 The disorder is characterized by a pattern of continued pathological use of a medication, non-medically indicated drug or toxin, that results in repeated adverse social consequences related to drug use, such as failure to meet work, family, or school obligations, interpersonal conflicts, or legal problems. There are on-going debates as to the exact distinctions between Substance abuse and substance dependence, but current practice standard distinguishes between the two by defining substance dependence in terms of physiological and behavioral symptoms of substance use, and Substance abuse in terms of the social consequences of substance use.
Huntington's disease	Huntington's disease is a neurodegenerative genetic disorder that affects muscle coordination and leads to cognitive decline and dementia. It typically becomes noticeable in middle age. Huntington's disease is the most common genetic cause of abnormal involuntary writhing movements called chorea.
Dyskinesia	Dyskinesia is a movement disorder which consists of effects including diminished voluntary movements and the presence of involuntary movements, similar to tics or chorea. Dyskinesia is a symptom of several medical disorders and is distinguished by the underlying cause.

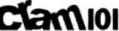

Chapter 9. Psychosis and Schizophrenia

Dystonia	Dystonia is a neurological movement disorder, in which sustained muscle contractions cause twisting and repetitive movements or abnormal postures. The disorder may be hereditary or caused by other factors such as birth-related or other physical trauma, infection, poisoning or reaction to pharmaceutical drugs, particularly neuroleptics.

· Generalized

· Focal

· Segmental

· Intermediate

· Acute Dystonic Reaction

· Normal birth history and milestones

· Autosomal dominant

· childhood onset

· starts in lower limbs and spreads upwards

· also known as 'idiopathic torsion Dystonia' (old terminology 'Dystonia musculrum deformans')
These are the most common Dystonias and tend to be classified as follows:

The combination of blepharospasmodic contractions and oromandibular Dystonia is called cranial Dystonia or Meige's syndrome.

Segmental Dystonias affect two adjoining parts of the body:

· HemiDystonia affects an arm and a leg on one side of the body.

· Multifocal Dystonia affects many different parts of the body.

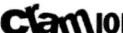

· Generalized Dystonia affects most of the body, frequently involving the legs and back.

There is a group called myoclonus Dystonia or myoclonic Dystonia, where some cases are hereditary and have been associated with a missense mutation in the dopamine-D2 receptor.

Tardive dyskinesia	Tardive dyskinesia is a variety of dyskinesia (involuntary, repetitive movements) manifesting as a side effect of long-term or high-dose use of dopamine antagonists, usually antipsychotics. Other dopamine antagonists that can cause Tardive dyskinesia are drugs for gastrointestinal disorders (e.g. metoclopramide) and neurological disorders. While newer atypical antipsychotics such as olanzapine and risperidone appear to have less dystonic effects, only clozapine has been shown to have a lower risk of Tardive dyskinesia than older antipsychotics.
Bipolar disorder	Bipolar disorder or manic-depressive disorder is a psychiatric diagnosis that describes a category of mood disorders defined by the presence of one or more episodes of abnormally elevated mood clinically referred to as mania or, if milder, hypomania. Individuals who experience manic episodes also commonly experience depressive episodes or symptoms, or mixed episodes in which features of both mania and depression are present at the same time. These episodes are usually separated by periods of 'normal' mood, but in some individuals, depression and mania may rapidly alternate, known as rapid cycling.
Prolixin	Fluphenazine is a typical antipsychotic drug used for the treatment of psychoses such as schizophrenia and acute manic phases of bipolar disorder. It belongs to the piperazine class of phenothiazines and is extremely potent; more potent than haloperidol and around fifty to seventy times the potency of chlorpromazine. It is marketed under the brand name of Prolixin and Sydocate(Surge Laboratories).
Amyloid	Amyloids are insoluble fibrous protein aggregates sharing specific structural traits. Abnormal accumulation of amyloid in organs may lead to amyloidosis, and may play a role in various neurodegenerative diseases. The name amyloid comes from the early mistaken identification of the substance as starch, based on crude iodine-staining techniques.

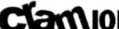

Chapter 9. Psychosis and Schizophrenia

Biosynthesis	Biosynthesis is an enzyme-catalyzed process in cells of living organisms by which substrates are converted to more complex products. The biosynthesis process often consists of several enzymatic steps in which the product of one step is used as substrate in the following step. Examples for such multi-step biosynthetic pathways are those for the production of amino acids, fatty acids, and natural products.
Pathophysiology	Pathophysiology is the study of the changes of normal mechanical, physical, and biochemical functions, either caused by a disease, or resulting from an abnormal syndrome. More formally, it is the branch of medicine which deals with any disturbances of body functions, caused by disease or prodromal symptoms. An alternative definition is 'the study of the biological and physical manifestations of disease as they correlate with the underlying abnormalities and physiological disturbances.' The study of pathology and the study of pathophysiology often involves substantial overlap in diseases and processes, but pathology emphasizes direct observations, while pathophysiology emphasizes quantifiable measurements.
Serotonin	Serotonin is a monoamine neurotransmitter. Biochemically derived from tryptophan, serotonin is primarily found in the gastrointestinal (GI) tract, platelets, and in the central nervous system (CNS) of animals including humans. It is a well-known contributor to feelings of well-being; therefore it is also known as a 'happiness hormone' despite not being a hormone.
Ketamine	Ketamine is a drug used in human and veterinary medicine developed by Parke-Davis (today a part of Pfizer) in 1962. Its hydrochloride salt is sold as Ketanest, Ketaset, and Ketalar. Pharmacologically, Ketamine is classified as an NMDA receptor antagonist.
Amino acid	Amino acids are molecules containing an amine group, a carboxylic acid group and a side-chain that varies between different amino acids. The key elements of an amino acid are carbon, hydrogen, oxygen, and nitrogen. They are particularly important in biochemistry, where the term usually refers to alpha-amino acids.
Estrogen	Estrogens (U.S., otherwise oEstrogens or Å"strogens) are a group of steroid compounds and functioning as the primary female sex hormone, their name comes from estrus/oistros (period of fertility for female mammals) + gen/gonos = to generate.

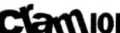

Chapter 9. Psychosis and Schizophrenia

	Estrogens are used as part of some oral contraceptives, in Estrogen replacement therapy for postmenopausal women, and in hormone replacement therapy for trans women.
	Like all steroid hormones, Estrogens readily diffuse across the cell membrane.
Glutamate receptors	Glutamate receptors are synaptic receptors located primarily on the membranes of neuronal cells. Glutamate is one of the 20 amino acids used to assemble proteins and as a result is abundant in many areas of the body, but it also functions as a neurotransmitter and is particularly abundant in the nervous system. Glutamate receptors are responsible for the glutamate-mediated post-synaptic excitation of neural cells, and are important for neural communication, memory formation, learning, and regulation.
Excitotoxicity	Excitotoxicity is the pathological process by which nerve cells are damaged and killed by glutamate and similar substances. This occurs when receptors for the excitatory neurotransmitter glutamate (glutamate receptors) such as the NMDA receptor and AMPA receptor are overactivated. Excitotoxins like NMDA and kainic acid which bind to these receptors, as well as pathologically high levels of glutamate, can cause Excitotoxicity by allowing high levels of calcium ions (Ca^{2+}) to enter the cell.
Antipsychotic	An antipsychotic is a tranquilizing psychiatric medication primarily used to manage psychosis (including delusions or hallucinations, as well as disordered thought), particularly in schizophrenia and bipolar disorder. A first generation of antipsychotics, known as typical antipsychotics, was discovered in the 1950s. Most of the drugs in the second generation, known as atypical antipsychotics, have been developed more recently, although the first atypical antipsychotic, clozapine, was discovered in the 1950s and introduced clinically in the 1970s.
Brain-derived neurotrophic factor	Brain-derived neurotrophic factor is a protein that, in humans, is encoded by the Brain derived neurotrophic factor gene. Brain derived neurotrophic factor is a member of the 'neurotrophin' family of growth factors, which are related to the canonical 'Nerve Growth Factor', NGF. Neurotrophic factors are found in the brain and the periphery.
Radicals	In chemistry, radicals are atoms, molecules, or ions with unpaired electrons on an open shell configuration. The unpaired electrons cause them to be highly chemically reactive. radicals play an important role in combustion, atmospheric chemistry, polymerization, plasma chemistry, biochemistry, and many other chemical processes, including human physiology.

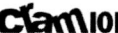

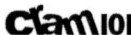

Chapter 9. Psychosis and Schizophrenia

Long-term potentiation	In neuroscience, Long-term potentiation is a long-lasting enhancement in signal transmission between two neurons that results from stimulating them synchronously. It is one of several phenomena underlying synaptic plasticity, the ability of chemical synapses to change their strength. As memories are thought to be encoded by modification of synaptic strength, LTP is widely considered one of the major cellular mechanisms that underlies learning and memory.

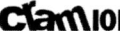

Chapter 10. Antipsychotic Agents

Rheumatology	Rheumatology is a sub-specialty in internal medicine and pediatrics, devoted to diagnosis and therapy of conditions and diseases affecting joints, muscles, and bones. Clinicians who specialize in rheumatology are called rheumatologists. Rheumatologists deal mainly with clinical problems involving joints, soft tissues, certain autoimmune diseases, vasculitis, and heritable connective tissue disorders.
Chlorpromazine	Chlorpromazine is the oldest typical antipsychotic. The molecular structure is 2-chloro-10-(3-dimethylaminopropyl)-phenothiazine. Chlorpromazine effectively treats schizophrenia, severe mania in people with bipolar disorder, and uncontrollable hiccups.
Chloride channels	Chloride channels are a superfamily of poorly understood ion channels consisting of approximately 13 members. Chloride channels display a variety of important physiological and cellular roles that include regulation of pH, volume homeostasis, organic solute transport, cell migration, cell proliferation and differentiation. Based on sequence homology the Chloride channels can be subdivided into a number of groups.
Fibromyalgia	Fibromyalgia is also referred to as FM or FMS. Fibromyalgia is characterized by chronic widespread pain and allodynia, a heightened and painful response to pressure.
Off-label use	Off-label use is the practice of prescribing pharmaceuticals for a purpose outside the scope of a drug's approved label - an unproven, untested use - most often concerning the drug's indication. In the United States, the Food and Drug Administration (FDA) requires numerous clinical trials to prove a drug's safety and efficacy in treating a given disease or condition. If satisfied that the drug is safe and effective, the drug's manufacturer and the FDA agree on specific language describing dosage, route and other information to be included on the drug's label.
Receptor	In biochemistry, a receptor is a protein molecule, embedded in either the plasma membrane or the cytoplasm of a cell, to which one or more specific kinds of signaling molecules may attach. A molecule which binds (attaches) to a receptor is called a ligand, and may be a peptide (short protein) or other small molecule, such as a neurotransmitter, a hormone, a pharmaceutical drug, or a toxin. Each kind of receptor can bind only certain ligand shapes.
Symptom	A Symptom is a departure from normal function or feeling which is noticed by a patient, indicating the presence of disease or abnormality. A Symptom is subjective, observed by the patient, and not measured.

Chapter 10. Antipsychotic Agents

Syndrome	In medicine and psychology, a Syndrome is the association of several clinically recognizable features, signs (observed by a physician), symptoms (reported by the patient), phenomena or characteristics that often occur together, so that the presence of one feature alerts the physician to the presence of the others. In recent decades, the term has been used outside medicine to refer to a combination of phenomena seen in association. The term Syndrome derives from its Greek roots and means literally 'run together', as the features do.
Psychopharmacology	Psychopharmacology is the study of drug-induced changes in mood, sensation, thinking, and behavior. The field of Psychopharmacology studies a wide range of substances with various types of psychoactive properties. The professional and commercial fields of pharmacology and Psychopharmacology do not mainly focus on psychedelic or recreational drugs, as the majority of studies are conducted for the development, study, and use of drugs for the modification of behavior and the alleviation of symptoms, particularly in the treatment of mental disorders .
Number needed to harm	The Number needed to harm (NNH) is an epidemiological measure that indicates how many patients need to be exposed to a risk-factor to cause harm in one patient that would not otherwise have been harmed. It is defined as the inverse of the attributable risk. Intuitively, the lower the Number needed to harm the worse the risk-factor.
Abuse	Abuse is defined as:
Addiction	The term 'addiction' is used in many contexts to describe an obsession, compulsion, or excessive psychological dependence, such as: drug addiction problem gambling, crime, money, work addiction, compulsive overeating, Oniomania (compulsive shopping), computer addiction, video game addiction, pornography addiction, television addiction, etc. In medical terminology, an addiction is a chronic neurobiologic disorder that has genetic, psychosocial, and environmental dimensions and is characterized by one of the following: the continued use of a substance despite its detrimental effects, impaired control over the use of a drug (compulsive behavior), and preoccupation with a drug's use for non-therapeutic purposes (i.e. craving the drug). addiction is often accompanied by the presence of deviant behaviors (for instance stealing money and forging prescriptions) that are used to obtain a drug.

Chapter 10. Antipsychotic Agents

Antipsychotic	An antipsychotic is a tranquilizing psychiatric medication primarily used to manage psychosis (including delusions or hallucinations, as well as disordered thought), particularly in schizophrenia and bipolar disorder. A first generation of antipsychotics, known as typical antipsychotics, was discovered in the 1950s. Most of the drugs in the second generation, known as atypical antipsychotics, have been developed more recently, although the first atypical antipsychotic, clozapine, was discovered in the 1950s and introduced clinically in the 1970s.
Bipolar disorder	Bipolar disorder or manic-depressive disorder is a psychiatric diagnosis that describes a category of mood disorders defined by the presence of one or more episodes of abnormally elevated mood clinically referred to as mania or, if milder, hypomania. Individuals who experience manic episodes also commonly experience depressive episodes or symptoms, or mixed episodes in which features of both mania and depression are present at the same time. These episodes are usually separated by periods of 'normal' mood, but in some individuals, depression and mania may rapidly alternate, known as rapid cycling.
Huntington's disease	Huntington's disease is a neurodegenerative genetic disorder that affects muscle coordination and leads to cognitive decline and dementia. It typically becomes noticeable in middle age. Huntington's disease is the most common genetic cause of abnormal involuntary writhing movements called chorea.
Dopamine	Dopamine is a neurotransmitter that occurs in a wide variety of animals, including both vertebrates and invertebrates. In the brain, this phenethylamine functions as a neurotransmitter, activating the five types of Dopamine receptors--D_1, D_2, D_3, D_4, and D_5--and their variants. Dopamine is produced in several areas of the brain, including the substantia nigra and the ventral tegmental area.
Hyperprolactinaemia	Hyperprolactinaemia is the presence of abnormally-high levels of prolactin in the blood. Normal levels are less than 500 mIU/L for women, and less than 450 mIU/L for men. Prolactin is a peptide hormone produced by the anterior pituitary gland primarily associated with lactation and plays a vital role in breast development during pregnancy. Hyperprolactinaemia may cause production and spontaneous flow of breast milk and disruptions in the normal menstrual period in women and hypogonadism, infertility and erectile dysfunction in men.
Cholinergic	A receptor is cholinergic if it uses acetylcholine as its neurotransmitter.

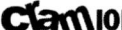

CRAM101

Chapter 10. Antipsychotic Agents

	cholinergic means related to the neurotransmitter acetylcholine, and is typically used in a neurological perspective. The parasympathetic nervous system is entirely cholinergic.
Constipation	Constipation, costiveness) experiences hard feces that is difficult to expel. This usually happens because the colon absorbs too much water from the food. If the food moves through the gastro-intestinal tract too slowly, the colon may absorb too much water, resulting in feces that are dry and hard.
Acetylcholine	The chemical compound Acetylcholine is a neurotransmitter in both the peripheral nervous system (PNS) and central nervous system (CNS) in many organisms including humans. Acetylcholine is one of many neurotransmitters in the autonomic nervous system (ANS) and the only neurotransmitter used in the motor division of the somatic nervous system. (Sensory neurons use glutamate and various peptides at their synapses).
Atrophy	Atrophy is the partial or complete wasting away of a part of the body. Causes of Atrophy include poor nourishment, poor circulation, loss of hormonal support, loss of nerve supply to the target organ, disuse or lack of exercise or disease intrinsic to the tissue itself. Hormonal and nerve inputs that maintain an organ or body part are referred to as trophic [noun] in medical practice.
Atypical antipsychotics	The Atypical antipsychotics are a group of antipsychotic drugs used to treat psychiatric conditions. Some Atypical antipsychotics are FDA approved for use in the treatment of schizophrenia. Some carry FDA approved indications for acute mania, bipolar mania, psychotic agitation, bipolar maintenance, and other indications.
Cardiovascular	The circulatory system is an organ system that passes nutrients (such as amino acids and electrolytes), gases, hormones, blood cells, etc. to and from cells in the body to help fight diseases and help stabilize body temperature and pH to maintain homeostasis. This system may be seen strictly as a blood distribution network, but some consider the circulatory system as composed of the cardiovascular system, which distributes blood, and the lymphatic system, which distributes lymph.
Glucocorticoid	Glucocorticoids (GC) are a class of steroid hormones that bind to the Glucocorticoid receptor (GR), which is present in almost every vertebrate animal cell. The name Glucocorticoid derives from their role in the regulation of the metabolism of glucose, their synthesis in the adrenal cortex, and their steroidal structure .
	GCs are part of the feedback mechanism in the immune system that turns immune activity (inflammation) down.

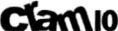

Chapter 10. Antipsychotic Agents

Norepinephrine	Noradrenaline (BAN) is a catecholamine with dual roles as a hormone and a neurotransmitter. As a stress hormone, Norepinephrine affects parts of the brain where attention and responding actions are controlled. Along with epinephrine, Norepinephrine also underlies the fight-or-flight response, directly increasing heart rate, triggering the release of glucose from energy stores, and increasing blood flow to skeletal muscle.
Side effect	In medicine, a side effect is an effect, whether therapeutic or adverse, that is secondary to the one intended; although the term is predominantly employed to describe adverse effects, it can also apply to beneficial, but unintended, consequences of the use of a drug. Occasionally, drugs are prescribed or procedures performed specifically for their side effects; in that case, said side effect ceases to be a side effect, and is now an intended effect. For instance, X-rays were historically (and are currently) used as an imaging technique; the discovery of their oncolytic capability led to their employ in radiotherapy (ablation of malignant tumours).
Agonist	An Agonist is a drug that binds to a receptor of a cell and triggers a response by the cell. An Agonist often mimics the action of a naturally occurring substance. An Agonist produces an action.
Neuroleptic malignant syndrome	Neuroleptic malignant syndrome is a life threatening, although rare neurological disorder most often caused by an adverse reaction to neuroleptic or antipsychotic drugs. It generally presents with muscle rigidity, fever, autonomic instability and cognitive changes such as delirium, and is associated with elevated creatine phosphokinase (CPK). Incidence of the disease has declined since its discovery (due to proactive prescription habits), but it is still dangerous to patients being treated with antipsychotics.
Schizophrenia	Schizophrenia , from the Greek roots skhizein and phrÄ"n, phren- (φρÎ®v, φρεv-; 'mind') is a psychiatric diagnosis that describes a neuropsychiatric and mental disorder characterized by abnormalities in the perception or expression of reality. It most commonly manifests as auditory hallucinations, paranoid or bizarre delusions, or disorganized speech and thinking with significant social or occupational dysfunction. Onset of symptoms typically occurs in young adulthood, with around 0.4-0.6% of the population affected.

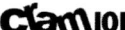

Chapter 10. Antipsychotic Agents

Serotonin	Serotonin is a monoamine neurotransmitter. Biochemically derived from tryptophan, serotonin is primarily found in the gastrointestinal (GI) tract, platelets, and in the central nervous system (CNS) of animals including humans. It is a well-known contributor to feelings of well-being; therefore it is also known as a 'happiness hormone' despite not being a hormone.
Amino acid	Amino acids are molecules containing an amine group, a carboxylic acid group and a side-chain that varies between different amino acids. The key elements of an amino acid are carbon, hydrogen, oxygen, and nitrogen. They are particularly important in biochemistry, where the term usually refers to alpha-amino acids.
Brain-derived neurotrophic factor	Brain-derived neurotrophic factor is a protein that, in humans, is encoded by the Brain derived neurotrophic factor gene. Brain derived neurotrophic factor is a member of the 'neurotrophin' family of growth factors, which are related to the canonical 'Nerve Growth Factor', NGF. Neurotrophic factors are found in the brain and the periphery.
Serotonin receptors	The serotonin receptors also known as 5-hydroxytryptamine receptors or 5-HT receptors are a group of G protein-coupled receptors (GPCRs) and ligand-gated ion channels (LGICs) found in the central and peripheral nervous systems. They mediate both excitatory and inhibitory neurotransmission. The serotonin receptors are activated by the neurotransmitter serotonin, which acts as their natural ligand.
Estrogen	Estrogens (U.S., otherwise oEstrogens or Å"strogens) are a group of steroid compounds and functioning as the primary female sex hormone, their name comes from estrus/oistros (period of fertility for female mammals) + gen/gonos = to generate.
	Estrogens are used as part of some oral contraceptives, in Estrogen replacement therapy for postmenopausal women, and in hormone replacement therapy for trans women.
	Like all steroid hormones, Estrogens readily diffuse across the cell membrane.
Extrapyramidal symptoms	The extrapyramidal system can be affected in a number of ways, which are revealed in a range of Extrapyramidal symptoms such as akinesia (inability to initiate movement) and akathisia (inability to remain motionless).

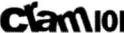

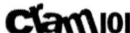

Chapter 10. Antipsychotic Agents

	Extrapyramidal symptoms are the various movement disorders such as tardive dyskinesia suffered as a result of taking dopamine antagonists, usually antipsychotic (neuroleptic) drugs, which are often used to control psychosis.
	The Simpson-Angus Scale (SAS) and the Barnes Akathisia Rating Scale (BARS) are used to measure Extrapyramidal symptoms.
Inverse agonist	In pharmacology, an Inverse agonist is an agent which binds to the same receptor binding-site as an agonist for that receptor and reverses constitutive activity of receptors. Inverse agonists exert the opposite pharmacological effect of a receptor agonist. Inverse agonists are effective against certain types of receptors (e.g. certain histamine receptors and GABA receptors) which have intrinsic activity without the action of a ligand upon them (also referred to as 'constitutive activity').
Anticholinergic	An Anticholinergic agent is a substance that blocks the neurotransmitter acetylcholine in the central and the peripheral nervous system. An example of an Anticholinergic is dicyclomine, and the classic example is atropine. Anticholinergics are administered to reduce the effects mediated by acetylcholine on acetylcholine receptors in neurons through competitive inhibition.
Anticholinergic	An Anticholinergic agent is a substance that blocks the neurotransmitter acetylcholine in the central and the peripheral nervous system. An example of an Anticholinergic is dicyclomine, and the classic example is atropine. Anticholinergics are administered to reduce the effects mediated by acetylcholine on acetylcholine receptors in neurons through competitive inhibition.
Deficiency	A Deficiency is a lack of something. Example
	there is a Deficiency of oxygen in the air and we shall soon suffocate.
	· In mathematics, a deficient number is a number n for which $\sigma(n) < 2n$.
	· In medicine there are a variety of nutrient deficiencies:
	· Avitaminosis is a Deficiency of vitamins.
	· Boron Deficiency
	· Chromium Deficiency

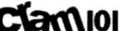

Chapter 10. Antipsychotic Agents

· Iron Deficiency

· Iodine Deficiency

· Magnesium Deficiency

· Micronutrient Deficiency

· In construction, a Deficiency is an item, or condition that is considered sub-standard, or below minimum expectations, such as those mandated by either drawings or specifications or the building code or the fire code, and/or any combination of the foregoing. Deficiencies are routinely discussed and dealt with in construction site meetings.

· In genetics, a genetic deletion is also called a Deficiency.

· In real estate law, a Deficiency in the ability to pay off a debt is called a Deficiency judgment or Deficiency judgement.

Huntington's disease	Huntington's disease is a neurodegenerative genetic disorder that affects muscle coordination and leads to cognitive decline and dementia. It typically becomes noticeable in middle age. Huntington's disease is the most common genetic cause of abnormal involuntary writhing movements called chorea.
Amyloid	Amyloids are insoluble fibrous protein aggregates sharing specific structural traits. Abnormal accumulation of amyloid in organs may lead to amyloidosis, and may play a role in various neurodegenerative diseases.
	The name amyloid comes from the early mistaken identification of the substance as starch, based on crude iodine-staining techniques.
Nicotinic	Nicotinic acetylcholine receptors, are cholinergic receptors that form ligand-gated ion channels in the plasma membranes of certain neurons. Being ionotropic receptors, nAChRs are directly linked to an ion channel and do not make use of a second messenger as metabotropic receptors do.

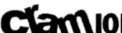

Chapter 10. Antipsychotic Agents

	Like the other type of acetylcholine receptors - muscarinic acetylcholine receptors (mAChRs) - the nAChR is triggered by the binding of the neurotransmitter acetylcholine (ACh).
Prolactin	Prolactin or Luteotropic hormone (LTH) is a peptide hormone discovered by Dr. Henry Friesen, primarily associated with lactation. In breastfeeding, the act of an infant suckling the nipple stimulates the production of Prolactin, which fills the breast with milk via a process called lactogenesis, in preparation for the next feed. Oxytocin, another hormone, is also released, which triggers milk let-down.
Secretion	Secretion is the process of elaborating, releasing, and oozing chemicals, or a secreted chemical substance from a cell or gland. In contrast to excretion, the substance may have a certain function, rather than being a waste product. Secretion in bacterial species means the transport or translocation of effector molecules for example proteins, enzymes or toxins (such as cholera toxin in pathogenic bacteria for example Vibrio cholerae) from across the interior (cytoplasm or cytosol) of a bacterial cell to its exterior.
Antihistamine	A histamine antagonist is an agent that serves to inhibit the release or action of histamine. antihistamine can be used to describe any histamine antagonist, but it is usually reserved for the classical antihistamines that act upon the H_1 histamine receptor. antihistamines are used as treatment for allergies.
Histidine	Histidine Histidine an essential amino acid, has a positively charged imidazole functional group. It is the one of the 22 proteinogenic amino acids. Its codons are CAU and CAC. Histidine was first isolated by German physician Albrecht Kossel in 1896. Histidine is an essential amino acid in humans and other mammals.
Benadryl	Benadryl is a brand name allergy medicine marketed over-the-counter by Johnson ' Johnson subsidiary McNeil Consumer Healthcare. Prior to 2007, Benadryl was marketed by Pfizer Consumer Healthcare. Benadryl is used as an antihistamine for the temporary relief of seasonal and perennial allergy symptoms.

Chapter 10. Antipsychotic Agents

Aripiprazole	Aripiprazole (ay-ri-PIP-ray-zole) (marketed as Abilify, Abilify Discmelt; also known as BMS 337039, OPC-14597, and APZ) was approved by the Food and Drug Administration (FDA) on November 15, 2002 for the treatment of schizophrenia, the sixth atypical antipsychotic medication of its kind. More recently, it received FDA approval for the treatment of acute manic and mixed episodes associated with bipolar disorder, and as an adjunct for the treatment of major depressive disorder. Aripiprazole was developed by Otsuka in Japan; in the U.S., Otsuka America markets the drug jointly with Bristol-Myers Squibb.
Bifeprunox	Bifeprunox is a novel atypical antipsychotic agent which, along with SLV313, aripiprazole, and SSR-181507 combines minimal D_2 receptor agonism with 5-HT receptor agonism.
	Bifeprunox has a novel mechanism of action. Conventional antipsychotics are classed into typical and atypical.
Interaction	Interaction is a kind of action that occurs as two or more objects have an effect upon one another. The idea of a two-way effect is essential in the concept of Interaction, as opposed to a one-way causal effect. A closely related term is interconnectivity, which deals with the Interactions of Interactions within systems: combinations of many simple Interactions can lead to surprising emergent phenomena.
Histamine	Histamine is a biogenic amine involved in local immune responses as well as regulating physiological function in the gut and acting as a neurotransmitter. Histamine triggers the inflammatory response. As part of an immune response to foreign pathogens, Histamine is produced by basophils and by mast cells found in nearby connective tissues.
Histamine receptors	The Histamine receptors are a class of G-protein coupled receptors with histamine as their endogenous ligand.
	There are four known Histamine receptors:
	· H_1 receptor
	· H_2 receptor
	· H_3 receptor
	· H_4 receptor

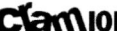

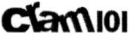

Chapter 10. Antipsychotic Agents

	There are several splice variants of H_3 present in various species. Though all of the receptors are 7-transmembrane g protein coupled receptors, H_1 and H_2 are quite different from H_3 and H_4 in their activities. H_1 causes an increase in PIP_2 hydrolysis, H2 stimulates gastric acid secretion, and H3 mediates feedback inhibition of histamine.
Insulin	insulin is a hormone that has extensive effects on metabolism and other body functions, such as vascular compliance. insulin causes cells in the liver, muscle, and fat tissue to take up glucose from the blood, storing it as glycogen in the liver and muscle, and stopping use of fat as an energy source. When insulin is absent (or low), glucose is not taken up by body cells, and the body begins to use fat as an energy source, for example, by transfer of lipids from adipose tissue to the liver for mobilization as an energy source.
Insulin resistance	Insulin resistance is a condition in which body cells become less sensitive to the glucose-lowering effects of the hormone insulin. In most cases in humans, normal blood levels of insulin become inadequate to keep blood glucose within a normal range. Not all cell types require insulin to absorb glucose, but the major groups which do include fat and muscle cells.
Sinequan	Doxepin is a psychotropic agent with tricyclic antidepressant and anxiolytic properties, known under many brand-names such as Aponal, the original preparation by Boehringer-Mannheim, now part of the Roche group; Adapine, Deptran, Sinquan and Sinequan . As doxepin hydrochloride, it is the active ingredient in cream-based preparations (Zonalon and Xepin) for the treatment of dermatological itch. Doxepin is currently investigated for the treatment of insomnia, and the proposed tradename of doxepin for this indication is Silenor.
Neurotransmitters	Neurotransmitters are endogenous chemicals which relay, amplify, and modulate signals between a neuron and another cell. Neurotransmitters are packaged into synaptic vesicles that cluster beneath the membrane on the presynaptic side of a synapse, and are released into the synaptic cleft, where they bind to receptors in the membrane on the postsynaptic side of the synapse. Release of Neurotransmitters usually follows arrival of an action potential at the synapse, but may follow graded electrical potentials.
Triglycerides	(more properly known as , TAG or triacylglyceride) is a glyceride in which the glycerol is esterified with three fatty acids. It is the main constituent of vegetable oil and animal fats. Triglycerides are formed from a single molecule of glycerol, combined with three fatty acids on each of the OH groups, and make up most of fats digested by humans.

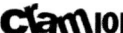

Clam101

Chapter 10. Antipsychotic Agents

Sedation	Sedation is a medical procedure involving the administration of sedative drugs, generally to facilitate a medical procedure or diagnostic proceedure. Drugs which can be used for Sedation include propofol, etomidate, ketamine, fentanyl and midazolam.
Cytochromes	Cytochromes are, in general, membrane-bound hemoproteins that contain heme groups and carry out electron transport. They are found either as monomeric proteins (e.g., cytochrome c) or as subunits of bigger enzymatic complexes that catalyze redox reactions. They are found in the mitochondrial inner membrane and endoplasmic reticulum of eukaryotes, in the chloroplasts of plants, in photosynthetic microorganisms, and in bacteria.
Cytochrome P450	The cytochrome P450 superfamily is a large and diverse group of enzymes. The function of most CYP enzymes is to catalyze the oxidation of organic substances. The substrates of CYP enzymes include metabolic intermediates such as lipids and steroidal hormones, as well as xenobiotic substances such as drugs and other toxic chemicals.
Enzyme	Enzymes are proteins that catalyze (i.e., increase the rates of) chemical reactions. In enzymatic reactions, the molecules at the beginning of the process are called substrates, and the Enzyme converts them into different molecules, called the products. Almost all processes in a biological cell need Enzymes to occur at significant rates.
Pharmacodynamics	Pharmacodynamics is the study of the physiological effects of drugs on the body or on microorganisms or parasites within or on the body and the mechanisms of drug action and the relationship between drug concentration and effect. One dominant example is drug-receptor interactions as modeled by $$L + R \leftrightarrow L \cdot R$$ where L=ligand (drug), R=receptor (attachment site), reaction dynamics that can be studied mathematically through tools such as free energy maps. Pharmacodynamics is often summarized as the study of what a drug does to the body, whereas pharmacokinetics is the study of what the body does to a drug.

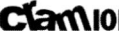

Chapter 10. Antipsychotic Agents

Pharmacokinetics	Pharmacokinetics is a branch of pharmacology dedicated to the determination of the fate of substances administered externally to a living organism. In practice, this discipline is applied mainly to drug substances, though in principle it concerns itself with all manner of compounds ingested or otherwise delivered externally to an organism, such as nutrients, metabolites, hormones, toxins, etc.
	pharmacokinetics is often studied in conjunction with pharmacodynamics.
Antidepressant	An antidepressant is a psychiatric medication used to alleviate mood disorders, such as major depression and dysthymia and anxiety disorders such as social anxiety disorder. According to Gelder, Mayou '*Geddes (2005) people with a depressive illness will experience a therapeutic effect to their mood, however this will not be experienced in healthy individuals. Drugs including the monoamine oxidase inhibitors (MAOIs), tricyclic antidepressants (TCAs), tetracyclic antidepressants (TeCAs), selective serotonin reuptake inhibitors (SSRIs), and serotonin-norepinephrine reuptake inhibitors (SNRIs) are most commonly associated with the term.
Insomnia	Insomnia is a symptom which can accompany several sleep, medical and psychiatric disorders, characterized by persistent difficulty falling asleep and/or staying asleep despite the opportunity. Insomnia is typically followed by functional impairment while awake. Both organic and non-organic Insomnia without other cause constitute a sleep disorder, primary Insomnia.
Zaleplon	Zaleplon is a sedative/hypnotic, mainly used for insomnia. It is a nonbenzodiazepine hypnotic from the pyrazolopyrimidine class. In terms of adverse effects Zaleplon appears to offer little improvement compared to both benzodiazepines and other non-benzodiazepine Z-drugs.
Ziprasidone	Ziprasidone was the fifth atypical antipsychotic to gain FDA approval (February 2001). In the United States, Ziprasidone is Food and Drug Administration (FDA) approved for the treatment of schizophrenia, and the intramuscular injection form of Ziprasidone is approved for acute agitation in schizophrenic patients. Ziprasidone has also received approval for acute treatment of mania and mixed states associated with bipolar disorder.
Zotepine	Zotepine is an atypical antipsychotic indicated for acute and chronic schizophrenia. It has been used in Germany since 1990 and Japan since 1982.
	The antipsychotic effect of Zotepine is thought to be mediated through antagonist activity at dopamine and serotonin receptors.

Chapter 10. Antipsychotic Agents

Clozapine	Clozapine is an antipsychotic medication used in the treatment of schizophrenia. The first of the atypical antipsychotics to be developed, it was first introduced in Europe in 1971, but was voluntarily withdrawn by the manufacturer in 1975 after it was shown to cause agranulocytosis, a condition involving a dangerous decrease in the number of white blood cells, that led to death in some patients. In 1989, after studies demonstrated that it was more effective than any other antipsychotic for treating schizophrenia, the U.S. Food and Drug Administration (FDA) approved Clozapine's use but only for treatment-resistant schizophrenia.
Seizure	An epileptic Seizure is a transient symptom of excessive or synchronous neuronal activity in the brain. It can manifest as an alteration in mental state, tonic or clonic movements, convulsions, and various other psychic symptoms (such as déjà vu or jamais vu). The medical syndrome of recurrent, unprovoked Seizures is termed epilepsy, but Seizures can occur in people who do not have epilepsy.
Prolixin	Fluphenazine is a typical antipsychotic drug used for the treatment of psychoses such as schizophrenia and acute manic phases of bipolar disorder. It belongs to the piperazine class of phenothiazines and is extremely potent; more potent than haloperidol and around fifty to seventy times the potency of chlorpromazine. It is marketed under the brand name of Prolixin and Sydocate(Surge Laboratories).
Fluoxetine	Fluoxetine (trade name Prozac) is an antidepressant of the selective serotonin reuptake inhibitor (SSRI) class. Fluoxetine is approved for the treatment of major depression (including pediatric depression), obsessive-compulsive disorder (in both adult and pediatric populations), bulimia nervosa, anorexia nervosa, panic disorder and premenstrual dysphoric disorder. Despite the availability of newer agents, it remains extremely popular.
Fluvoxamine	Fluvoxamine is an antidepressant which functions as a selective serotonin reuptake inhibitor (SSRI). Fluvoxamine was first approved by the U.S. Food and Drug Administration (FDA) in 1993 for the treatment of obsessive compulsive disorder (OCD). Fluvoxamine CR (controlled release) is approved to treat social anxiety disorder.
Ketoconazole	Ketoconazole is a synthetic antifungal drug used to prevent and treat skin and fungal infections, especially in immunocompromised patients such as those with AIDS. Ketoconazole is sold commercially as an anti-dandruff shampoo, topical cream, and oral tablet, under the trademark name Nizoral by Johnson ' Johnson.
	Ketoconazole is very lipophilic, which leads to accumulation in fatty tissues. The less toxic and more effective triazole compounds fluconazole and itraconazole have largely replaced Ketoconazole for internal use.

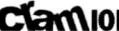

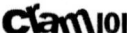

Chapter 10. Antipsychotic Agents

Protease	A protease is any enzyme that conducts proteolysis, that is, begins protein catabolism by hydrolysis of the peptide bonds that link amino acids together in the polypeptide chain forming the protein.
	Proteases are currently classified into six broad groups:
	<ul><li>Serine proteases</li><li>Threonine proteases</li><li>Cysteine proteases</li><li>Aspartate proteases</li><li>Metalloproteases</li><li>Glutamic acid proteases</li></ul>
	The threonine and glutamic-acid proteases were not described until 1995 and 2004, respectively. The mechanism used to cleave a peptide bond involves making an amino acid residue that has the cysteine and threonine (proteases) or a water molecule (aspartic acid, metallo- and glutamic acid proteases) nucleophilic so that it can attack the peptide carboxyl group.
Protease inhibitors	Researchers are investigating the use of protease inhibitors developed for HIV treatment as anti-protozoals for use against malaria and gastrointestinal protozoal infections:
	· A combination of ritonavir and lopinavir was found to have some effectiveness against Giardia infection.
	· The drugs saquinavir, ritonavir, and lopinavir have been found to have anti-malarial properties.
	· A cysteine protease inhibitor drug was found to cure Chagas disease in mice. Researchers are investigating whether protease inhibitors could possibly be used to treat cancer. For example, nelfinavir and atazanavir are able to kill tumor cells in culture (in a Petri dish).

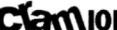

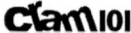

Chapter 10. Antipsychotic Agents

Mood stabilizer	A Mood stabilizer is a psychiatric medication used to treat mood disorders characterized by intense and sustained mood shifts, which is not the same as 'feeling good one minute and then bad the next.' One use is in bipolar disorder, where Mood stabilizers suppress swings between mania and depression. These drugs are also used in borderline personality disorder. Most Mood stabilizers are purely antimanic agents, meaning that they are effective at treating mania and mood cycling and shifting, but are not effective at treating depression.
Drug interaction	A Drug interaction is a situation in which a substance affects the activity of a drug, i.e. the effects are increased or decreased, or they produce a new effect that neither produces on its own. Typically, interaction between drugs come to mind (drug-Drug interaction). However, interactions may also exist between drugs ' foods (drug-food interactions), as well as drugs ' herbs (drug-herb interactions).
Aventyl	Nortriptyline is a second-generation tricyclic antidepressant marketed as the hydrochloride under the trade names Sensoval, Aventyl, Pamelor, Norpress, Allegron and Nortrilen. It is used in the treatment of major depression and childhood nocturnal enuresis (bedwetting). In addition, it is sometimes used for chronic illnesses such as chronic fatigue syndrome, chronic pain and migraines, and labile affect in some neurological conditions.
Agranulocytosis	Agranulocytosis, also known as agranulosis, is an acute condition involving a severe and dangerous leukopenia (lowered white blood cell count), most commonly of neutrophils, causing a neutropenia in the circulating blood. It represents a severe lack of one major class of infection-fighting white blood cells. People with this condition are at very high risk of serious infections due to their suppressed immune system.
Olanzapine	Olanzapine is an atypical antipsychotic, approved by the FDA for the treatment of schizophrenia and bipolar disorder. The Olanzapine formulations are manufactured and marketed by the pharmaceutical company Eli Lilly and Company, whose patent f proper expires in 2011 (in October 2009 a Canadian judge ruled that the 1991 patent was invalid). Sales of Zyprexa in 2008 were $2.2B in the US alone, and $4.7B in total.

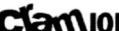

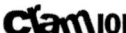

· oral formulation: acute and maintenance treatment of Schizophrenia in adults, acute treatment of manic or mixed episodes associated with Bipolar I Disorder (monotherapy and in combination with lithium or valproate)

· intramuscular formulation: acute agitation associated with Schizophrenia and Bipolar I Mania in adults

· oral formulation combined with fluoxetine: acute treatment of depressive episodes associated with Bipolar I Disorder in adults, or acute treatment of treatment resistant depression in adults
Known FDA approvals are as follows:

· approved for the treatment of the manifestations of psychotic disorders on September 6, 1996

· approved in combination with fluoxetine for the treatment of depressive episodes associated with Bipolar disorder on December 24, 2003

· approved for the long-term treatment of bipolar I disorder on January 14, 2004

· approved in combination with fluoxetine for treatment resistant depression on March 19, 2009. Off-label uses are listed below.

Amitriptyline	Amitriptyline is a psychoactive drug and pharmaceutical of the tricyclic antidepressant (TCA) chemical class which is used primarily as an antidepressant and anxiolytic agent. It is the most widely prescribed TCA and perhaps also the most efficient against depressive symptoms.
	Amitriptyline is approved for the treatment of major depression.

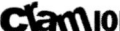

CTam101

Chapter 10. Antipsychotic Agents

Psychosis	Psychosis means abnormal condition of the mind, and is a generic psychiatric term for a mental state often described as involving a 'loss of contact with reality'. People suffering from Psychosis are said to be psychotic. People experiencing Psychosis may report hallucinations or delusional beliefs, and may exhibit personality changes and thought disorder.
Risperidone	Risperidone is an atypical antipsychotic used to treat schizophrenia , the mixed and manic states associated with bipolar disorder, and irritability in children with autism. The drug was developed by Janssen-Cilag and first released in 1994. It is sold under the trade name Risperdal in the Netherlands, United States, Canada, the United Kingdom, Portugal, Spain, Turkey, New Zealand and several other countries, Risperdal or Ridal in New Zealand, Sizodon or Riscalin in India, Rispolept in Eastern Europe, and Belivon, or Rispen elsewhere. · treatment of schizophrenia in adults · treatment of schizophrenia in adolescents aged 13-17 years · alone or in combination with lithium or valproate, for the short-term treatment of acute manic or mixed episodes associated with Bipolar I Disorder in adults · alone the short-term treatment of acute manic or mixed episodes associated with Bipolar I Disorder in children and adolescents aged 10-17 years · treatment of irritability associated with autistic disorder in children and adolescents aged 5-16 years Risperidone was approved by the United States Food and Drug Administration (FDA) in 1993 for the treatment of schizophrenia. On August 22, 2007, Risperdal was approved as the only drug agent available for treatment of schizophrenia in youth ages 13-17; it was also approved that same day for treatment of bipolar disorder in youth and children ages 10-17, joining lithium.

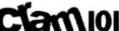

Chapter 10. Antipsychotic Agents

Norpramin	Desipramine is a tricyclic antidepressant (TCA) that inhibits the reuptake of norepinephrine and serotonin and to a lesser extent dopamine. It is sold under the brand names Norpramin and Pertofrane. It is used to treat depression, but not considered a first line treatment since the introduction of SSRI antidepressants.
Quetiapine	Quetiapine fumarate , marketed by AstraZeneca as Seroquel or SeroquelXR and by Orion Pharma as Ketipinor, is an atypical antipsychotic used in the management of schizophrenia, bipolar I mania, bipolar II depression, bipolar I depression, and used off-label for a variety of other purposes, including insomnia and anxiety disorders. Annual sales are approx. $4.7bn worldwide, and $2.9bn in the US. The US patent, which was set to expire in 2011, received a pediatric exclusivity extension which pushed its expiration to March 26, 2012; however, in Canada it has already expired.
Carbamazepine	Carbamazepine (CBZ) is an anticonvulsant and mood stabilizing drug used primarily in the treatment of epilepsy and bipolar disorder, as well as trigeminal neuralgia. It is also used off-label for a variety of indications, including attention-deficit hyperactivity disorder (ADHD), schizophrenia, phantom limb syndrome, paroxysmal extreme pain disorder, and post-traumatic stress disorder. Carbamazepine was discovered by chemist Walter Schindler at J.R. Geigy AG (now part of Novartis) in Basel, Switzerland, in 1953.
Infarction	In medicine, an infarction is the formation of an infarct, that is, an area of tissue death (necrosis) due to a local lack of oxygen caused by obstruction of the tissue's blood supply. The supplying artery may be blocked by an obstruction (e.g. an arterial embolus, thrombus, or atherosclerotic plaque), may be mechanically compressed (e.g. tumor, volvulus, or hernia), ruptured by trauma (e.g. atherosclerosis or vasculitides), or vasoconstricted (e.g. cocaine vasoconstriction leading to myocardial infarction).
Myocardial infarction	Myocardial infarction commonly known as a heart attack, is the interruption of blood supply to part of the heart, causing some heart cells to die. This is most commonly due to occlusion (blockage) of a coronary artery following the rupture of a vulnerable atherosclerotic plaque, which is an unstable collection of lipids (fatty acids) and white blood cells (especially macrophages) in the wall of an artery. The resulting ischemia (restriction in blood supply) and oxygen shortage, if left untreated for a sufficient period of time, can cause damage or death (infarction) of heart muscle tissue (myocardium).

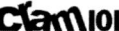

Chapter 10. Antipsychotic Agents

Asenapine	Asenapine (Saphris) is a new atypical antipsychotic developed for the treatment of schizophrenia and acute mania associated with bipolar disorder by Schering-Plough after its November 19, 2007 merge with Organon International. Development of the drug, through Phase III trials, began while Organon was still a part of Akzo Nobel. Preliminary data indicate that it has minimal anticholinergic and cardiovascular side effects, as well as minimal weight gain.
Loxapine	Loxapine is a typical antipsychotic medication, used primarily in the treatment of schizophrenia. It is a member of the dibenzoxazepine class and as a dibenzazepine derivative, it is structurally related to clozapine (which belongs to the chemically closely akin class of dibenzodiazepines). Several researchers have argued that Loxapine may behave as an atypical antipsychotic.
Akathisia	Akathisia, or acathisia, is a syndrome characterized by unpleasant sensations of 'inner' restlessness that manifests itself with an inability to sit still or remain motionless . Its most common cause is as a side effect of medications, mainly neuroleptic antipsychotics especially the phenothiazines , thioxanthenes (such as flupenthixol and zuclopenthixol) and butyrophenones (such as haloperidol (Haldol)), piperazines (such as ziprasidone), antispasmodics (such as metoclopramide), and antidepressants. Akathisia can also, to a lesser extent, be caused by Parkinson's disease and related syndromes.
Clinical trials	Clinical trials are conducted to allow safety and efficacy data to be collected for new drugs or devices. These trials can only take place once satisfactory information has been gathered on the quality of the product and its non-clinical safety, and Health Authority/Ethics Committee approval is granted in the country where the trial is taking place. Depending on the type of product and the stage of its development, investigators enroll healthy volunteers and/or patients into small pilot studies initially, followed by larger scale studies in patients that often compare the new product with the currently prescribed treatment.
Narcolepsy	Narcolepsy is a chronic sleep disorder, or dyssomnia. The condition is characterized by excessive daytime sleepiness (EDS) in which a person experiences extreme fatigue and possibly falls asleep at inappropriate times, such as while at work or at school. A narcoleptic will most likely experience disturbed nocturnal sleep and also abnormal daytime sleep pattern, which is often confused with insomnia.
First line treatment	A First-line treatment or first-line therapy is a medical therapy recommended for the initial treatment of a disease, sign or symptom, usually on the basis of empirical evidence for its efficacy.

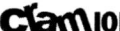

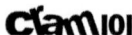

Chapter 10. Antipsychotic Agents

This evidence, often based on scientific research studies, of which the randomized controlled trial is the gold standard, typically suggests the recommended therapy is most likely to have an effect for the given condition.

Alternative treatment options, including switching to another treatment, or augmenting the First-line treatment with another treatment, may be recommended if the first-line therapy does not ease the symptoms, or produces intolerable side effects.

Injection

An injection is an infusion method of putting fluid into the body, usually with a hollow needle and a syringe which is pierced through the skin to a sufficient depth for the material to be forced into the body. An injection follows a parenteral route of administration, that is, administered other than through the digestive tract.

There are several methods of injection or infusion, including intradermal, subcutaneous, intramuscular, intravenous, intraosseous, and intraperitoneal.

Pharmacy

Pharmacy is the health profession that links the health sciences with the chemical sciences and it is charged with ensuring the safe and effective use of pharmaceutical drugs.

The scope of pharmacy practice includes more traditional roles such as compounding and dispensing medications, and it also includes more modern services related to health care, including clinical services, reviewing medications for safety and efficacy, and providing drug information. Pharmacists, therefore, are the experts on drug therapy and are the primary health professionals who optimize medication use to provide patients with positive health outcomes.

Stroke

A Stroke is the rapidly developing loss of brain function(s) due to disturbance in the blood supply to the brain. This can be due to ischemia (lack of glucose ' oxygen supply) caused by thrombosis or embolism or due to a hemorrhage. As a result, the affected area of the brain is unable to function, leading to inability to move one or more limbs on one side of the body, inability to understand or

The traditional definition of Stroke, devised by the World Health Organization in the 1970s, is a 'neurological deficit of cerebrovascular cause that persists beyond 24 hours or is interrupted by death within 24 hours'.

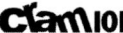

Cram101

Chapter 10. Antipsychotic Agents

Dementia	Dementia is a serious cognitive disorder. It may be static, the result of a unique global brain injury or progressive, resulting in long-term decline in cognitive function due to damage or disease in the body beyond what might be expected from normal aging. Although Dementia is far more common in the geriatric population, it may occur in any stage of adulthood.
Titration	Titration, is a common laboratory method of quantitative chemical analysis that is used to determine the unknown concentration of a known reactant. Because volume measurements play a key role in titration, it is also known as volumetric analysis. A reagent, called the titrant or titrator, of a known concentration (a standard solution) and volume is used to react with a solution of the analyte or titrand, whose concentration is not known.
Polypharmacy	The term polypharmacy generally refers to the use of multiple medications by a patient. The term is used when too many forms of medication are used by a patient, when more drugs are prescribed than is clinically warranted, or even when all prescribed medications are clinically indicated but there are too many pills to take (pill burden). Furthermore, a portion of the treatments may not be evidence-based.
Amantadine	Amantadine is the organic compound known formally as 1-aminoadamantane. The molecule consists of adamantane backbone that is substituted at one of the four methyne positions with an amino group. This compound is sold under the name 'Symmetrel' for use both as an antiviral and an antiparkinsonian drug.
Calcium	Calcium is the chemical element with the symbol Ca and atomic number 20. It has an atomic mass of 40.078 amu. Calcium is a soft gray alkaline earth metal, and is the fifth most abundant element by mass in the Earth's crust. Calcium is also the fifth most abundant dissolved ion in seawater by both molarity and mass, after sodium, chloride, magnesium, and sulfate.
Calcium channel	A Calcium channel is an ion channel which displays selective permeabiltiy to calcium ions. It is sometimes synonymous as voltage-dependent Calcium channel, although there are also ligand-gated Calcium channels. The following tables explain gating, gene, location and function of different types of Calcium channels, both voltage and ligand-gated. · the receptor-operated Calcium channels (in vasoconstriction) · P2X receptor

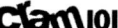

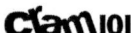

Chapter 10. Antipsychotic Agents

	Calcium channel blockers are used to treat hypertension.
Memantine	Memantine is the first in a novel class of Alzheimer's disease medications acting on the glutamatergic system by blocking NMDA glutamate receptors. Memantine is marketed under the brands Axura and Akatinol by Merz, Namenda by Forest, Ebixa and Abixa by Lundbeck and Memox by Unipharm. Although Memantine is approved for treatment of moderate to severe Alzheimer's disease, its usage has been recommended against by the UK's National Institute for Clinical Excellence, on the grounds that its high cost outweighs the benefits of treatment in most patients.
Pharmacology	Pharmacology is the study of drug action. More specifically, it is the study of the interactions that occur between a living organism and exogenous chemicals that alter normal biochemical function. If substances have medicinal properties, they are considered pharmaceuticals.
Galantamine	Galantamine is a chemical used for the treatment of mild to moderate Alzheimer's disease and various memory impairments. It is an alkaloid that is obtained synthetically or from the bulbs and flowers of the Caucasian snowdrop (Voronov's snowdrop), Galanthus woronowii (Amaryllidaceae) and related genera like Narcissus (daffodil), Leucojum (snowflake) and Lycoris including Lycoris radiata (Red Spider Lily). The active ingredient was isolated by prof.
Mirtazapine	Mirtazapine is a psychoactive drug of the benzazepine and tetracyclic antidepressant (TeCA) chemical classes which is used primarily as an antidepressant. It is sometimes used for its anxiolytic, hypnotic, antiemetic, orexigenic, and antihistamine or antipruritic effects. Mirtazapine was introduced by Organon International in 1994. Along with its chemical analogue and predecessor mianserin (Bolvidon, Norval, Tolvon), Mirtazapine is one of the few noradrenergic and specific serotonergic antidepressants (NaSSAs).
Buspirone	Buspirone is a psychoactive drug and pharmaceutical medication of the piperazine and azapirone chemical classes. It is used primarily as an anxiolytic, but also to a lesser extent as an antidepressant. Bristol-Myers Squibb (BMS) gained Food and Drug Administration (FDA) approval for Buspirone in 1986, and it went generic in 2001.

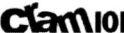

Cl̶am̶\101

Chapter 10. Antipsychotic Agents

Cannabinoid	Cannabinoids are a group of terpenophenolic compounds present in Cannabis (Cannabis sativa L) and which occur naturally in the nervous and immune systems of animals. The broader definition of Cannabinoids refers to a group of substances that are structurally related to tetrahydrocannabinol (THC) or that bind to Cannabinoid receptors. The chemical definition encompasses a variety of distinct chemical classes: the classical Cannabinoids structurally related to THC, the nonclassical Cannabinoids, the aminoalkylindoles, the eicosanoids related to the endoCannabinoids, 1,5-diarylpyrazoles, quinolines and arylsulphonamides and additional compounds that do not fall into these standard classes but bind to Cannabinoid receptors.
Rimonabant	Rimonabant is an anorectic anti-obesity drug. It is an inverse agonist for the cannabinoid receptor CB1. Its main avenue of effect is reduction in appetite. Rimonabant was the first selective CB1 receptor blocker to be approved for use anywhere in the world.
Varenicline	Varenicline is a prescription medication used to treat smoking addiction. Varenicline is a nicotinic receptor partial agonist. In this respect, it is similar to cytisine and different from the nicotinic antagonist, bupropion, and nicotine replacement therapies (NRTs) like nicotine patches (commonly, 'the patch') and nicotine gum.
Antibiotic	In common usage, an Antibiotic is a substance or compound that kills, or inhibits the growth of, bacteria. Antibiotics belong to the broader group of antimicrobial compounds, used to treat infections caused by microorganisms, including fungi and protozoa. The term 'Antibiotic' was coined by Selman Waksman in 1942 to describe any substance produced by a microorganism that is antagonistic to the growth of other microorganisms in high dilution.
Atorvastatin	Atorvastatin is a member of the drug class known as statins, used for lowering blood cholesterol. It also stabilizes plaque and prevents strokes through anti-inflammatory and other mechanisms.

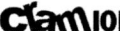

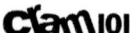

Chapter 10. Antipsychotic Agents

	Atorvastatin inhibits HMG-CoA reductase, the rate-determining enzyme located in hepatic tissue that produces mevalonate, a small molecule used in the synthesis of cholesterol and other mevalonate derivatives. This lowers the amount of cholesterol produced which in turn lowers the total amount of LDL cholesterol. Atorvastatin was first synthesized in 1985 by Bruce Roth while working at Parke-Davis Warner-Lambert Company (now Pfizer).
Erythromycin	Erythromycin is a macrolide antibiotic that has an antimicrobial spectrum similar to or slightly wider than that of penicillin, and is often used for people who have an allergy to penicillins. For respiratory tract infections, it has better coverage of atypical organisms, including mycoplasma and Legionellosis. It was first marketed by Eli Lilly and Company, and it is today commonly known as EES (Erythromycin ethylsuccinate, an ester prodrug that is commonly administered).
Macrolide	The macrolides are a group of drugs (typically antibiotics) whose activity stems from the presence of a macrolide ring, a large macrocyclic lactone ring to which one or more deoxy sugars, usually cladinose and desosamine, may be attached. The lactone rings are usually 14, 15 or 16-membered. macrolides belong to the polyketide class of natural products.

· Azithromycin (Zithromax, Zitromax, Sumamed, Azitrox) - Unique, does not inhibit CYP3A4

· Clarithromycin (Biaxin, Fromilid, Klacid, Klabax, Lekoklar)

· Dirithromycin (Dynabac)

· Erythromycin

· Roxithromycin (Rulid, Surlid, Roxid)

· Telithromycin

· Carbomycin A

· Josamycin

· Kitasamycin

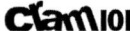

Chapter 10. Antipsychotic Agents

· Midecamicine/midecamicine acetate

· Oleandomycin

· Spiramycin

· Troleandomycin

· Tylosin/tylocine (Tylan)

Ketolides are a new class of antibiotics that are structurally related to the macrolides.

Peptide	Peptides are short polymers formed from the linking, in a defined order, of α-amino acids. The link between one amino acid residue and the next is called an amide bond or a Peptide bond. Proteins are polyPeptide molecules, or consist of multiple polyPeptide subunits, each composed of chains containing a specific sequence of the 22 proteinogenic amino acids.
Simvastatin	Simvastatin is a hypolipidemic drug belonging to the class of pharmaceuticals called 'statins'. It is used to control hypercholesterolemia (elevated cholesterol levels) and to prevent cardiovascular disease. Simvastatin is a synthetic derivate of a fermentation product of Aspergillus terreus.
Triazolam	Triazolam is a benzodiazepine derivative drug. It possesses pharmacological properties similar to that of other benzodiazepines, but it is generally only used as a sedative to treat insomnia. In addition to the hypnotic properties Triazolam possesses, amnesic, anxiolytic, sedative, anticonvulsant and muscle relaxant properties are also present.

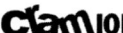

Chapter 11. Mood Disorders

Abuse	Abuse is defined as:
Cocaine	Cocaine is a crystalline tropane alkaloid that is obtained from the leaves of the coca plant. The name comes from 'coca' in addition to the alkaloid suffix -ine, forming Cocaine. It is a stimulant of the central nervous system and an appetite suppressant.
Neurotransmitters	Neurotransmitters are endogenous chemicals which relay, amplify, and modulate signals between a neuron and another cell. Neurotransmitters are packaged into synaptic vesicles that cluster beneath the membrane on the presynaptic side of a synapse, and are released into the synaptic cleft, where they bind to receptors in the membrane on the postsynaptic side of the synapse. Release of Neurotransmitters usually follows arrival of an action potential at the synapse, but may follow graded electrical potentials.
Norepinephrine	Noradrenaline (BAN) is a catecholamine with dual roles as a hormone and a neurotransmitter. As a stress hormone, Norepinephrine affects parts of the brain where attention and responding actions are controlled. Along with epinephrine, Norepinephrine also underlies the fight-or-flight response, directly increasing heart rate, triggering the release of glucose from energy stores, and increasing blood flow to skeletal muscle.
Benadryl	Benadryl is a brand name allergy medicine marketed over-the-counter by Johnson ' Johnson subsidiary McNeil Consumer Healthcare. Prior to 2007, Benadryl was marketed by Pfizer Consumer Healthcare. Benadryl is used as an antihistamine for the temporary relief of seasonal and perennial allergy symptoms.
Psychopharmacology	Psychopharmacology is the study of drug-induced changes in mood, sensation, thinking, and behavior.
	The field of Psychopharmacology studies a wide range of substances with various types of psychoactive properties. The professional and commercial fields of pharmacology and Psychopharmacology do not mainly focus on psychedelic or recreational drugs, as the majority of studies are conducted for the development, study, and use of drugs for the modification of behavior and the alleviation of symptoms, particularly in the treatment of mental disorders .

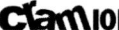

Chapter 11. Mood Disorders

Antidepressant	An antidepressant is a psychiatric medication used to alleviate mood disorders, such as major depression and dysthymia and anxiety disorders such as social anxiety disorder. According to Gelder, Mayou '*Geddes (2005) people with a depressive illness will experience a therapeutic effect to their mood, however this will not be experienced in healthy individuals. Drugs including the monoamine oxidase inhibitors (MAOIs), tricyclic antidepressants (TCAs), tetracyclic antidepressants (TeCAs), selective serotonin reuptake inhibitors (SSRIs), and serotonin-norepinephrine reuptake inhibitors (SNRIs) are most commonly associated with the term.
Huntington's disease	Huntington's disease is a neurodegenerative genetic disorder that affects muscle coordination and leads to cognitive decline and dementia. It typically becomes noticeable in middle age. Huntington's disease is the most common genetic cause of abnormal involuntary writhing movements called chorea.
Fibromyalgia	Fibromyalgia is also referred to as FM or FMS. Fibromyalgia is characterized by chronic widespread pain and allodynia, a heightened and painful response to pressure.
Mania	Mania is a state of abnormally elevated or irritable mood, arousal, and/ or energy levels, which is a criterion for certain psychiatric diagnoses; usually, it is a form of clinical psychosis. There are several possible causes f outside of mood disorders, including drug abuse and brain tumors, but it is most often associated with bipolar disorder, where episodes of Mania alternate with episodes of major depression. These cycles may relate to diurnal rhythms and environmental stressors.
Receptor	In biochemistry, a receptor is a protein molecule, embedded in either the plasma membrane or the cytoplasm of a cell, to which one or more specific kinds of signaling molecules may attach. A molecule which binds (attaches) to a receptor is called a ligand, and may be a peptide (short protein) or other small molecule, such as a neurotransmitter, a hormone, a pharmaceutical drug, or a toxin. Each kind of receptor can bind only certain ligand shapes.
Symptom	A Symptom is a departure from normal function or feeling which is noticed by a patient, indicating the presence of disease or abnormality. A Symptom is subjective, observed by the patient, and not measured.
Huntington's disease	Huntington's disease is a neurodegenerative genetic disorder that affects muscle coordination and leads to cognitive decline and dementia. It typically becomes noticeable in middle age. Huntington's disease is the most common genetic cause of abnormal involuntary writhing movements called chorea.

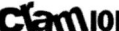

Chapter 11. Mood Disorders

Insomnia	Insomnia is a symptom which can accompany several sleep, medical and psychiatric disorders, characterized by persistent difficulty falling asleep and/or staying asleep despite the opportunity. Insomnia is typically followed by functional impairment while awake. Both organic and non-organic Insomnia without other cause constitute a sleep disorder, primary Insomnia.
Schizophrenia	Schizophrenia , from the Greek roots skhizein and phrÄ"n, phren- (φρÎ®ν, φρεν-; 'mind') is a psychiatric diagnosis that describes a neuropsychiatric and mental disorder characterized by abnormalities in the perception or expression of reality. It most commonly manifests as auditory hallucinations, paranoid or bizarre delusions, or disorganized speech and thinking with significant social or occupational dysfunction. Onset of symptoms typically occurs in young adulthood, with around 0.4-0.6% of the population affected.
Syndrome	In medicine and psychology, a Syndrome is the association of several clinically recognizable features, signs (observed by a physician), symptoms (reported by the patient), phenomena or characteristics that often occur together, so that the presence of one feature alerts the physician to the presence of the others. In recent decades, the term has been used outside medicine to refer to a combination of phenomena seen in association. The term Syndrome derives from its Greek roots and means literally 'run together', as the features do.
Schizoaffective disorder	Schizoaffective disorder is a psychiatric diagnosis that describes a mental disorder characterized by recurring episodes of elevated or depressed mood, or of simultaneously elevated and depressed mood, that alternate with, or occur together with, distortions in perception. Schizoaffective disorder most commonly affects cognition and emotion. Auditory hallucinations, paranoia, bizarre delusions, or disorganized speech and thinking with significant social and occupational dysfunction are typical.

Chapter 11. Mood Disorders

Bipolar disorder	Bipolar disorder or manic-depressive disorder is a psychiatric diagnosis that describes a category of mood disorders defined by the presence of one or more episodes of abnormally elevated mood clinically referred to as mania or, if milder, hypomania. Individuals who experience manic episodes also commonly experience depressive episodes or symptoms, or mixed episodes in which features of both mania and depression are present at the same time. These episodes are usually separated by periods of 'normal' mood, but in some individuals, depression and mania may rapidly alternate, known as rapid cycling.
Algorithm	In mathematics, computer science, and related subjects, an Algorithm is an effective method for solving a problem using a finite sequence of instructions. Algorithms are used for calculation, data processing, and many other fields. Each Algorithm is a list of well-defined instructions for completing a task.
Dopamine	Dopamine is a neurotransmitter that occurs in a wide variety of animals, including both vertebrates and invertebrates. In the brain, this phenethylamine functions as a neurotransmitter, activating the five types of Dopamine receptors--D_1, D_2, D_3, D_4, and D_5--and their variants. Dopamine is produced in several areas of the brain, including the substantia nigra and the ventral tegmental area.
Enzyme	Enzymes are proteins that catalyze (i.e., increase the rates of) chemical reactions. In enzymatic reactions, the molecules at the beginning of the process are called substrates, and the Enzyme converts them into different molecules, called the products. Almost all processes in a biological cell need Enzymes to occur at significant rates.
Interaction	Interaction is a kind of action that occurs as two or more objects have an effect upon one another. The idea of a two-way effect is essential in the concept of Interaction, as opposed to a one-way causal effect. A closely related term is interconnectivity, which deals with the Interactions of Interactions within systems: combinations of many simple Interactions can lead to surprising emergent phenomena.
Mirtazapine	Mirtazapine is a psychoactive drug of the benzazepine and tetracyclic antidepressant (TeCA) chemical classes which is used primarily as an antidepressant. It is sometimes used for its anxiolytic, hypnotic, antiemetic, orexigenic, and antihistamine or antipruritic effects. Mirtazapine was introduced by Organon International in 1994. Along with its chemical analogue and predecessor mianserin (Bolvidon, Norval, Tolvon), Mirtazapine is one of the few noradrenergic and specific serotonergic antidepressants (NaSSAs).

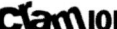

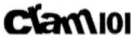

Chapter 11. Mood Disorders

Noradrenaline	Noradrenaline or norepinephrine (INN) is a catecholamine with dual roles as a hormone and a neurotransmitter.
	As a stress hormone, norepinephrine affects parts of the brain where attention and responding actions are controlled. Along with epinephrine, norepinephrine also underlies the fight-or-flight response, directly increasing heart rate, triggering the release of glucose from energy stores, and increasing blood flow to skeletal muscle.
Tyramine	Tyramine is a naturally-occurring monoamine compound and trace amine derived from the amino acid tyrosine. Tyramine acts as a catecholamine (dopamine, norepinephrine (noradrenaline), epinephrine (adrenaline)) releasing agent. Notably, however, it is unable to cross the blood-brain-barrier (BBB), resulting in only non-psychoactive peripheral sympathomimetic effects.
Serotonin	Serotonin is a monoamine neurotransmitter. Biochemically derived from tryptophan, serotonin is primarily found in the gastrointestinal (GI) tract, platelets, and in the central nervous system (CNS) of animals including humans. It is a well-known contributor to feelings of well-being; therefore it is also known as a 'happiness hormone' despite not being a hormone.
Antihistamine	A histamine antagonist is an agent that serves to inhibit the release or action of histamine. antihistamine can be used to describe any histamine antagonist, but it is usually reserved for the classical antihistamines that act upon the H_1 histamine receptor.
	antihistamines are used as treatment for allergies.
Histidine	Histidine Histidine an essential amino acid, has a positively charged imidazole functional group. It is the one of the 22 proteinogenic amino acids. Its codons are CAU and CAC. Histidine was first isolated by German physician Albrecht Kossel in 1896. Histidine is an essential amino acid in humans and other mammals.
Cerebrospinal fluid	Cerebrospinal fluid Liquor cerebrospinalis, is a clear bodily fluid that occupies the subarachnoid space and the ventricular system around and inside the brain. In essence, the brain 'floats' in it.
	The CSF occupies the space between the arachnoid mater (the middle layer of the brain cover, meninges), and the pia mater (the layer of the meninges closest to the brain).

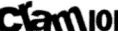

Chapter 11. Mood Disorders

Mood stabilizer	A Mood stabilizer is a psychiatric medication used to treat mood disorders characterized by intense and sustained mood shifts, which is not the same as 'feeling good one minute and then bad the next.'
	One use is in bipolar disorder, where Mood stabilizers suppress swings between mania and depression.
	These drugs are also used in borderline personality disorder.
	Most Mood stabilizers are purely antimanic agents, meaning that they are effective at treating mania and mood cycling and shifting, but are not effective at treating depression.
Atrophy	Atrophy is the partial or complete wasting away of a part of the body. Causes of Atrophy include poor nourishment, poor circulation, loss of hormonal support, loss of nerve supply to the target organ, disuse or lack of exercise or disease intrinsic to the tissue itself. Hormonal and nerve inputs that maintain an organ or body part are referred to as trophic [noun] in medical practice.
Glucocorticoid	Glucocorticoids (GC) are a class of steroid hormones that bind to the Glucocorticoid receptor (GR), which is present in almost every vertebrate animal cell. The name Glucocorticoid derives from their role in the regulation of the metabolism of glucose, their synthesis in the adrenal cortex, and their steroidal structure .
	GCs are part of the feedback mechanism in the immune system that turns immune activity (inflammation) down.
Bradykinin	Bradykinin is a peptide that causes blood vessels to enlarge (dilate), and therefore causes blood pressure to lower. A class of drugs called ACE inhibitors, which are used to lower blood pressure, increase Bradykinin further lowering blood pressure. Bradykinin works on blood vessels through the release of prostacyclin, nitric oxide, and Endothelium-Derived Hyperpolarizing Factor.
First-line treatment	A First-line treatment or first-line therapy is a medical therapy recommended for the initial treatment of a disease, sign or symptom, usually on the basis of empirical evidence for its efficacy.
	This evidence, often based on scientific research studies, of which the randomized controlled trial is the gold standard, typically suggests the recommended therapy is most likely to have an effect for the given condition.

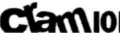

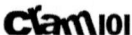
	Alternative treatment options, including switching to another treatment, or augmenting the First-line treatment with another treatment, may be recommended if the first-line therapy does not ease the symptoms, or produces intolerable side effects.
Citalopram	Citalopram is an antidepressant drug used to treat major depression associated with mood disorders. It is also used on occasion in the treatment of body dysmorphic disorder and anxiety. Citalopram belongs to a class of drugs known as selective serotonin reuptake inhibitors (SSRIs).
Eszopiclone	Eszopiclone, marketed by Sepracor under the brand-name Lunesta, is a nonbenzodiazepine hypnotic agent (viz., a sedative) used as a treatment for insomnia. Eszopiclone is the active stereoisomer of zopiclone, and belongs to the class of drugs known as cyclopyrrolones. Eszopiclone is a short acting nonbenzodiazepine sedative hypnotic.
Zopiclone	Zopiclone, (brand name Imovane in Canada, and Zimovane in the UK) is a non-benzodiazepine hypnotic agent used in the treatment of insomnia. In the United States, Zopiclone is not commercially available, although its active stereoisomer, esZopiclone, is sold under the names Lunesta . Zopiclone is a controlled substance in the United States, Canada, Japan, Brazil and some European countries, and may be illegal to possess without a prescription.

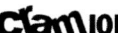

Cram101

Chapter 12. Antidepressants

Placebo	A placebo is a sham medical intervention. In one common placebo procedure, a patient is given an inert sugar pill, told that it may improve his/her condition, but not told that it is in fact inert. Such an intervention may cause the patient to believe the treatment will change his/her condition; and this belief does indeed sometimes have a therapeutic effect, causing the patient's condition to improve.
Tyramine	Tyramine is a naturally-occurring monoamine compound and trace amine derived from the amino acid tyrosine. Tyramine acts as a catecholamine (dopamine, norepinephrine (noradrenaline), epinephrine (adrenaline)) releasing agent. Notably, however, it is unable to cross the blood-brain-barrier (BBB), resulting in only non-psychoactive peripheral sympathomimetic effects.
Amitriptyline	Amitriptyline is a psychoactive drug and pharmaceutical of the tricyclic antidepressant (TCA) chemical class which is used primarily as an antidepressant and anxiolytic agent. It is the most widely prescribed TCA and perhaps also the most efficient against depressive symptoms. Amitriptyline is approved for the treatment of major depression.
Lewy bodies	Lewy bodies are abnormal aggregates of protein that develop inside nerve cells in Parkinson's disease (PD) and some other disorders. They are identified under the microscope when histology is performed on the brain. Lewy bodies appear as spherical masses that displace other cell components.
Antidepressant	An antidepressant is a psychiatric medication used to alleviate mood disorders, such as major depression and dysthymia and anxiety disorders such as social anxiety disorder. According to Gelder, Mayou '*Geddes (2005) people with a depressive illness will experience a therapeutic effect to their mood, however this will not be experienced in healthy individuals. Drugs including the monoamine oxidase inhibitors (MAOIs), tricyclic antidepressants (TCAs), tetracyclic antidepressants (TeCAs), selective serotonin reuptake inhibitors (SSRIs), and serotonin-norepinephrine reuptake inhibitors (SNRIs) are most commonly associated with the term.
Cholinergic	A receptor is cholinergic if it uses acetylcholine as its neurotransmitter. cholinergic means related to the neurotransmitter acetylcholine, and is typically used in a neurological perspective. The parasympathetic nervous system is entirely cholinergic.

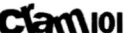

Chapter 12. Antidepressants

Acetylcholine	The chemical compound Acetylcholine is a neurotransmitter in both the peripheral nervous system (PNS) and central nervous system (CNS) in many organisms including humans. Acetylcholine is one of many neurotransmitters in the autonomic nervous system (ANS) and the only neurotransmitter used in the motor division of the somatic nervous system. (Sensory neurons use glutamate and various peptides at their synapses).
Amphetamine	Amphetamine (amfetamine (INN)) is a psychostimulant drug that is known to produce increased wakefulness and focus in association with decreased fatigue and appetite. Amphetamine is related to drugs such as methAmphetamine and dextroAmphetamine, which are a group of potent drugs that act by increasing levels of dopamine and norepinephrine in the brain, inducing euphoria. The group includes prescription CNS drugs commonly used to treat attention-deficit hyperactivity disorder (ADHD).
Mania	Mania is a state of abnormally elevated or irritable mood, arousal, and/ or energy levels, which is a criterion for certain psychiatric diagnoses; usually, it is a form of clinical psychosis. There are several possible causes f outside of mood disorders, including drug abuse and brain tumors, but it is most often associated with bipolar disorder, where episodes of Mania alternate with episodes of major depression. These cycles may relate to diurnal rhythms and environmental stressors.
Receptor	In biochemistry, a receptor is a protein molecule, embedded in either the plasma membrane or the cytoplasm of a cell, to which one or more specific kinds of signaling molecules may attach. A molecule which binds (attaches) to a receptor is called a ligand, and may be a peptide (short protein) or other small molecule, such as a neurotransmitter, a hormone, a pharmaceutical drug, or a toxin. Each kind of receptor can bind only certain ligand shapes.
Symptom	A Symptom is a departure from normal function or feeling which is noticed by a patient, indicating the presence of disease or abnormality. A Symptom is subjective, observed by the patient, and not measured.
Dopamine	Dopamine is a neurotransmitter that occurs in a wide variety of animals, including both vertebrates and invertebrates. In the brain, this phenethylamine functions as a neurotransmitter, activating the five types of Dopamine receptors--D_1, D_2, D_3, D_4, and D_5--and their variants. Dopamine is produced in several areas of the brain, including the substantia nigra and the ventral tegmental area.

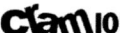

Chapter 12. Antidepressants

Syndrome	In medicine and psychology, a Syndrome is the association of several clinically recognizable features, signs (observed by a physician), symptoms (reported by the patient), phenomena or characteristics that often occur together, so that the presence of one feature alerts the physician to the presence of the others. In recent decades, the term has been used outside medicine to refer to a combination of phenomena seen in association. The term Syndrome derives from its Greek roots and means literally 'run together', as the features do.
Opioid	An opioid is a chemical that works by binding to opioid receptors, which are found principally in the central nervous system and the gastrointestinal tract. The receptors in these two organ systems mediate both the beneficial effects and the side effects of opioids. The analgesic effects of opioids are due to decreased perception of pain, decreased reaction to pain as well as increased pain tolerance.
Peptide	Peptides are short polymers formed from the linking, in a defined order, of α-amino acids. The link between one amino acid residue and the next is called an amide bond or a Peptide bond. Proteins are polyPeptide molecules, or consist of multiple polyPeptide subunits, each composed of chains containing a specific sequence of the 22 proteinogenic amino acids.
Serotonin	Serotonin is a monoamine neurotransmitter. Biochemically derived from tryptophan, serotonin is primarily found in the gastrointestinal (GI) tract, platelets, and in the central nervous system (CNS) of animals including humans. It is a well-known contributor to feelings of well-being; therefore it is also known as a 'happiness hormone' despite not being a hormone.
Side effect	In medicine, a side effect is an effect, whether therapeutic or adverse, that is secondary to the one intended; although the term is predominantly employed to describe adverse effects, it can also apply to beneficial, but unintended, consequences of the use of a drug.

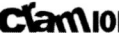

Chapter 12. Antidepressants

Occasionally, drugs are prescribed or procedures performed specifically for their side effects; in that case, said side effect ceases to be a side effect, and is now an intended effect. For instance, X-rays were historically (and are currently) used as an imaging technique; the discovery of their oncolytic capability led to their employ in radiotherapy (ablation of malignant tumours).

Tolerance	Toleration and Tolerance are terms used in social, cultural and religious contexts to describe attitudes which are 'tolerant' (or moderately respectful) of practices or group memberships that may be disapproved of by those in the majority. In practice, 'Tolerance' indicates support for practices that prohibit ethnic and religious discrimination. Conversely, 'inTolerance' may be used to refer to the discriminatory practices sought to be prohibited.
Deficiency	A Deficiency is a lack of something. Example

there is a Deficiency of oxygen in the air and we shall soon suffocate.

· In mathematics, a deficient number is a number n for which $\sigma(n) < 2n$.

· In medicine there are a variety of nutrient deficiencies:

· Avitaminosis is a Deficiency of vitamins.

· Boron Deficiency

· Chromium Deficiency

· Iron Deficiency

· Iodine Deficiency

· Magnesium Deficiency

· Micronutrient Deficiency

· In construction, a Deficiency is an item, or condition that is considered sub-standard, or below minimum expectations, such as those mandated by either drawings or specifications or the building code or the fire code, and/or any combination of the foregoing. Deficiencies are routinely discussed and dealt with in construction site meetings.

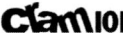

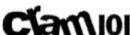

Chapter 12. Antidepressants

	· In genetics, a genetic deletion is also called a Deficiency.
	· In real estate law, a Deficiency in the ability to pay off a debt is called a Deficiency judgment or Deficiency judgement.
Norepinephrine	Noradrenaline (BAN) is a catecholamine with dual roles as a hormone and a neurotransmitter.
	As a stress hormone, Norepinephrine affects parts of the brain where attention and responding actions are controlled. Along with epinephrine, Norepinephrine also underlies the fight-or-flight response, directly increasing heart rate, triggering the release of glucose from energy stores, and increasing blood flow to skeletal muscle.
Diarrhea	In medicine, Diarrhea , also spelled diarrhoea , is the condition of having frequent loose or liquid bowel movements. Acute Diarrhea is a common cause of death in developing countries and the second most common cause of infant deaths worldwide. The loss of fluids through Diarrhea can cause severe dehydration which is one cause of death in Diarrhea sufferers.
Myoclonus	Myoclonus is brief, involuntary twitching of a muscle or a group of muscles. It describes a medical sign and, generally, is not a diagnosis of a disease. Brief twitches are perfectly normal.
Narcolepsy	Narcolepsy is a chronic sleep disorder, or dyssomnia. The condition is characterized by excessive daytime sleepiness (EDS) in which a person experiences extreme fatigue and possibly falls asleep at inappropriate times, such as while at work or at school. A narcoleptic will most likely experience disturbed nocturnal sleep and also abnormal daytime sleep pattern, which is often confused with insomnia.
Neurotransmitters	Neurotransmitters are endogenous chemicals which relay, amplify, and modulate signals between a neuron and another cell. Neurotransmitters are packaged into synaptic vesicles that cluster beneath the membrane on the presynaptic side of a synapse, and are released into the synaptic cleft, where they bind to receptors in the membrane on the postsynaptic side of the synapse. Release of Neurotransmitters usually follows arrival of an action potential at the synapse, but may follow graded electrical potentials.
Pharmacology	Pharmacology is the study of drug action. More specifically, it is the study of the interactions that occur between a living organism and exogenous chemicals that alter normal biochemical function. If substances have medicinal properties, they are considered pharmaceuticals.

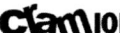

Chapter 12. Antidepressants

Serotonin receptors	The serotonin receptors also known as 5-hydroxytryptamine receptors or 5-HT receptors are a group of G protein-coupled receptors (GPCRs) and ligand-gated ion channels (LGICs) found in the central and peripheral nervous systems. They mediate both excitatory and inhibitory neurotransmission. The serotonin receptors are activated by the neurotransmitter serotonin, which acts as their natural ligand.
Vomiting	Vomiting is the forceful expulsion of the contents of one's stomach through the mouth and sometimes the nose. Vomiting may result from many causes, ranging from gastritis or poisoning to brain tumors, or elevated intracranial pressure. The feeling that one is about to vomit is called nausea, which usually precedes, but does not always lead to, Vomiting.
Psychopharmacology	Psychopharmacology is the study of drug-induced changes in mood, sensation, thinking, and behavior.
	The field of Psychopharmacology studies a wide range of substances with various types of psychoactive properties. The professional and commercial fields of pharmacology and Psychopharmacology do not mainly focus on psychedelic or recreational drugs, as the majority of studies are conducted for the development, study, and use of drugs for the modification of behavior and the alleviation of symptoms, particularly in the treatment of mental disorders .
Fluoxetine	Fluoxetine (trade name Prozac) is an antidepressant of the selective serotonin reuptake inhibitor (SSRI) class. Fluoxetine is approved for the treatment of major depression (including pediatric depression), obsessive-compulsive disorder (in both adult and pediatric populations), bulimia nervosa, anorexia nervosa, panic disorder and premenstrual dysphoric disorder. Despite the availability of newer agents, it remains extremely popular.
Half-life	Half-life is the period of time it takes for a substance undergoing decay to decrease by half. The name was originally used to describe a characteristic of unstable atoms (radioactive decay), but may apply to any quantity which follows a set-rate decay.
	The original term, dating to 1907, was 'Half-life period', which was later shortened to 'Half-life' in the early 1950s.
Sertraline	Sertraline hydrochloride (trade names Zoloft, Lustral) is an antidepressant of the selective serotonin reuptake inhibitor (SSRI) class. It was introduced to the market by Pfizer in 1991. Sertraline is primarily used to treat major depression in adult outpatients as well as obsessive-compulsive, panic, and social anxiety disorders in both adults and children. In 2007, it was the most prescribed antidepressant on the U.S. retail market, with 29,652,000 prescriptions.

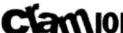

Chapter 12. Antidepressants

Tranylcypromine	Tranylcypromine is a psychoactive drug of the phenethylamine and amphetamine chemical classes which acts as a monoamine oxidase inhibitor (MAOI)--it is a nonselective and irreversible inhibitor of the enzyme monoamine oxidase (MAO). It is used as an antidepressant and anxiolytic agent in the clinical treatment of mood and anxiety disorders, respectively. Tranylcypromine is indicated primarily for the treatment of major depression without melancholia.
Paroxetine	Paroxetine is a selective serotonin reuptake inhibitor (SSRI) antidepressant. Marketing of the drug began in 1992 by the pharmaceutical company SmithKline Beecham, now GlaxoSmithKline. Paroxetine is used to treat major depression, obsessive-compulsive, panic, social anxiety, and generalised anxiety disorders in adult outpatients.
Fluvoxamine	Fluvoxamine is an antidepressant which functions as a selective serotonin reuptake inhibitor (SSRI). Fluvoxamine was first approved by the U.S. Food and Drug Administration (FDA) in 1993 for the treatment of obsessive compulsive disorder (OCD). Fluvoxamine CR (controlled release) is approved to treat social anxiety disorder.
Withdrawal	Withdrawal can refer to any sort of separation, but is most commonly used to describe the group of symptoms that occurs upon the abrupt discontinuation/separation or a decrease in dosage of the intake of medications, recreational drugs and/or alcohol. In order to experience the symptoms of withdrawal, one must have first developed a physical dependence (often referred to as chemical dependency). This happens after consuming one or more of these substances for a certain period of time, which is both dose dependent and varies based upon the drug consumed.
Citalopram	Citalopram is an antidepressant drug used to treat major depression associated with mood disorders. It is also used on occasion in the treatment of body dysmorphic disorder and anxiety. Citalopram belongs to a class of drugs known as selective serotonin reuptake inhibitors (SSRIs).
Eszopiclone	Eszopiclone, marketed by Sepracor under the brand-name Lunesta, is a nonbenzodiazepine hypnotic agent (viz., a sedative) used as a treatment for insomnia. Eszopiclone is the active stereoisomer of zopiclone, and belongs to the class of drugs known as cyclopyrrolones. Eszopiclone is a short acting nonbenzodiazepine sedative hypnotic.

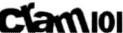

Chapter 12. Antidepressants

Hormone	A hormone is a chemical released by one or more cells that affects cells in other parts of the organism. Only a small amount of hormone is required to alter cell metabolism. It is essentially a chemical messenger that transports a signal from one cell to another.
Zopiclone	Zopiclone, (brand name Imovane in Canada, and Zimovane in the UK) is a non-benzodiazepine hypnotic agent used in the treatment of insomnia. In the United States, Zopiclone is not commercially available, although its active stereoisomer, esZopiclone, is sold under the names Lunesta . Zopiclone is a controlled substance in the United States, Canada, Japan, Brazil and some European countries, and may be illegal to possess without a prescription.
Escitalopram	Escitalopram (trade names Lexapro, Cipralex) is an antidepressant of the selective serotonin reuptake inhibitor (SSRI) class. It is approved by the U.S. Food and Drug Administration (FDA) for the treatment of major depressive disorder and generalized anxiety disorder in adults; other indications include social anxiety disorder, panic disorder and obsessive-compulsive disorder. Escitalopram is the S-stereoisomer (enantiomer) of the earlier Lundbeck drug citalopram (Celexa), hence the name Escitalopram.
Estrogen	Estrogens (U.S., otherwise oEstrogens or Å"strogens) are a group of steroid compounds and functioning as the primary female sex hormone, their name comes from estrus/oistros (period of fertility for female mammals) + gen/gonos = to generate.
	Estrogens are used as part of some oral contraceptives, in Estrogen replacement therapy for postmenopausal women, and in hormone replacement therapy for trans women.
	Like all steroid hormones, Estrogens readily diffuse across the cell membrane.
Dirty drug	A Dirty drug is an informal term used in pharmacology to describe drugs that may bind to many different molecular targets or receptors in the body, and so tend to have a wide range of effects and possibly negative side effects. Today, pharmaceutical companies try to make new drugs as selective as possible to minimise the occurrence of side effects and risk of adverse reactions. Examples of compounds often cited as 'Dirty drugs' include chlorpromazine, dextromethorphan and ibogaine, all of which bind to multiple receptors or influence multiple receptor systems.

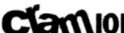

Chapter 12. Antidepressants

Tricyclic	tricyclic antidepressants (TCAs) are a class of psychoactive drugs used primarily as antidepressants, which were first discovered in the early 1950s, and subsequently introduced later in the decade. They are named after their chemical structure, which contains three rings of atoms. The 'tetracyclic antidepressants' (TeCAs), which contain four rings of atoms, are a closely related group that is often grouped together with the tricyclics, because clinically these drugs are primarily classified by their effect upon receptors.
Tricyclic antidepressants	tricyclic antidepressants are a class of psychoactive drugs used primarily as antidepressants, which were first discovered in the early 1950s, and subsequently introduced later in the decade. They are named after their chemical structure, which contains three rings of atoms. The 'tetracyclic antidepressants' (TeCAs), which contain four rings of atoms, are a closely related group that is often grouped together with the tricyclics, because clinically these drugs are primarily classified by their effect upon receptors.
Dopaminergic	Dopaminergic means related to the neurotransmitter dopamine. For example, certain proteins such as the dopamine transporter (DAT), vesicular monoamine transporter 2 (VMAT$_2$), and dopamine receptors can be classified as Dopaminergic, and neurons which synthesize or contain dopamine and synapses with dopamine receptors in them may also be labeled as Dopaminergic. Enzymes which regulate the biosynthesis or metabolism of dopamine such as aromatic L-amino acid decarboxylase (AAAD) or DOPA decarboxylase (DDC), monoamine oxidase (MAO), and catechol O-methyl transferase (COMT) may be referred to as Dopaminergic as well.
Schizophrenia	Schizophrenia , from the Greek roots skhizein and phrÄ"n, phren- (φρÎ®ν, φρεν-; 'mind') is a psychiatric diagnosis that describes a neuropsychiatric and mental disorder characterized by abnormalities in the perception or expression of reality. It most commonly manifests as auditory hallucinations, paranoid or bizarre delusions, or disorganized speech and thinking with significant social or occupational dysfunction. Onset of symptoms typically occurs in young adulthood, with around 0.4-0.6% of the population affected.
Anticholinergic	An Anticholinergic agent is a substance that blocks the neurotransmitter acetylcholine in the central and the peripheral nervous system. An example of an Anticholinergic is dicyclomine, and the classic example is atropine. Anticholinergics are administered to reduce the effects mediated by acetylcholine on acetylcholine receptors in neurons through competitive inhibition.

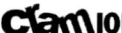

Chapter 12. Antidepressants

Antipsychotic	An antipsychotic is a tranquilizing psychiatric medication primarily used to manage psychosis (including delusions or hallucinations, as well as disordered thought), particularly in schizophrenia and bipolar disorder. A first generation of antipsychotics, known as typical antipsychotics, was discovered in the 1950s. Most of the drugs in the second generation, known as atypical antipsychotics, have been developed more recently, although the first atypical antipsychotic, clozapine, was discovered in the 1950s and introduced clinically in the 1970s.
Huntington's disease	Huntington's disease is a neurodegenerative genetic disorder that affects muscle coordination and leads to cognitive decline and dementia. It typically becomes noticeable in middle age. Huntington's disease is the most common genetic cause of abnormal involuntary writhing movements called chorea.
Protriptyline	Protriptyline is a tricyclic antidepressant (TCA), specifically a secondary amine, indicated for the treatment of depression and ADHD. Unique among the TCAs, Protriptyline tends to be energizing instead of sedating, and is sometimes used for narcolepsy to achieve a wakefulness-promoting effect. TCAs including Protriptyline are also used to reduce the incidence of recurring headaches such as migraine, and for other types of chronic pain. This drug can also be used for sleep apnea treatment along with a carbonic anhydrase inhibitor.
Urinary	The urinary system (also called excretory system or the genitourinary system) is the organ system that produces, stores, and eliminates urine. In humans it includes two kidneys, two ureters, the bladder, the urethra, and the penis in males. The analogous organ in invertebrates is the nephridium.
Venlafaxine	Venlafaxine is an arylalkanolamine serotonin-norepinephrine reuptake inhibitor (SNRI). First introduced by Wyeth in 1993, it is licensed for the treatment of major depressive disorder (MDD), as an anxiolytic, and comorbid indications. In 2007, Venlafaxine was the sixth most commonly prescribed antidepressant on the U.S. retail market, with 17.2 million prescriptions.
Desvenlafaxine	Desvenlafaxine, also known as O-desmethylvenlafaxine, is an antidepressant of the serotonin-norepinephrine reuptake inhibitor class developed and marketed by Wyeth (now part of Pfizer). Desvenlafaxine is a synthetic form of the major active metabolite of venlafaxine (Effexor, Efexor). It is being targeted as the first non-hormonal based treatment for menopause.

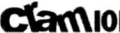

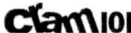

Chapter 12. Antidepressants

Risperidone	Risperidone is an atypical antipsychotic used to treat schizophrenia , the mixed and manic states associated with bipolar disorder, and irritability in children with autism. The drug was developed by Janssen-Cilag and first released in 1994. It is sold under the trade name Risperdal in the Netherlands, United States, Canada, the United Kingdom, Portugal, Spain, Turkey, New Zealand and several other countries, Risperdal or Ridal in New Zealand, Sizodon or Riscalin in India, Rispolept in Eastern Europe, and Belivon, or Rispen elsewhere. · treatment of schizophrenia in adults · treatment of schizophrenia in adolescents aged 13-17 years · alone or in combination with lithium or valproate, for the short-term treatment of acute manic or mixed episodes associated with Bipolar I Disorder in adults · alone the short-term treatment of acute manic or mixed episodes associated with Bipolar I Disorder in children and adolescents aged 10-17 years · treatment of irritability associated with autistic disorder in children and adolescents aged 5-16 years Risperidone was approved by the United States Food and Drug Administration (FDA) in 1993 for the treatment of schizophrenia. On August 22, 2007, Risperdal was approved as the only drug agent available for treatment of schizophrenia in youth ages 13-17; it was also approved that same day for treatment of bipolar disorder in youth and children ages 10-17, joining lithium.
Anxiety disorder	Anxiety disorder is a blanket term covering several different forms of abnormal and pathological fear and anxiety which only came under the aegis of psychiatry at the very end of the 19th century. Current psychiatric diagnostic criteria recognize a wide variety of Anxiety disorders. Recent surveys have found that as many as 18% of Americans may be affected by one or more of them.
Huntington's disease	Huntington's disease is a neurodegenerative genetic disorder that affects muscle coordination and leads to cognitive decline and dementia. It typically becomes noticeable in middle age. Huntington's disease is the most common genetic cause of abnormal involuntary writhing movements called chorea.

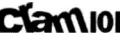

Chapter 12. Antidepressants

Duloxetine	Duloxetine is a serotonin-norepinephrine reuptake inhibitor manufactured and marketed by Eli Lilly. It is effective for major depressive disorder and it is as effective as venlafaxine in generalized anxiety disorder. Duloxetine failed the US approval for stress urinary incontinence amidst the concerns about liver toxicity and suicidal events; however, it was approved for this indication in Europe and Canada.
Chronic pain	Chronic pain has several different meanings in medicine. Traditionally, the distinction between acute and chronic pain has relied upon an arbitrary interval of time from onset; the two most commonly used markers being 3 months and 6 months since the initiation of pain, though some theorists and researchers have placed the transition from acute to chronic pain at 12 months. Others apply acute to pain that lasts less than 30 days, chronic to pain of more than six months duration, and subacute to pain that lasts from one to six months.
Sibutramine	Sibutramine, usually available as Sibutramine hydrochloride monohydrate, is an orally administered agent for the treatment of obesity, as an appetite suppressant. Serious concerns are being expressed about its safety and has been suspended from use in the UK and EU. It is also under review by the FDA and the European Medicines Agency. It is a centrally-acting serotonin-norepinephrine reuptake inhibitor structurally related to amphetamines, although its mechanism of action is distinct.
Affective spectrum	The affective spectrum is a grouping of related psychiatric and medical disorders which may accompany bipolar, unipolar, and schizoaffective disorders at statistically higher rates than would normally be expected. These disorders are identified by a common positive response to the same types of pharmacologic treatments. They also aggregate strongly in families and may therefore share common heritable underlying physiologic anomalies.
Bupropion	Bupropion previously known as amfebutamone, is an atypical antidepressant and smoking cessation aid. It acts as a strong norepinephrine and weak dopamine reuptake inhibitor, as well as $\alpha_3\beta_4$-nicotinic receptor antagonist. Bupropion belongs to the chemical class of aminoketones and is similar in structure to cathinone and diethylpropion, and to phenethylamines in general.
Atomoxetine	Atomoxetine is a drug approved for the treatment of attention-deficit hyperactivity disorder (ADHD). It is sold in the form of the hydrochloride salt of Atomoxetine, a norepinephrine reuptake inhibitor. This compound is manufactured, marketed and sold in the United States under the brand name Strattera by Eli Lilly and Company, the original patent filing company, and current U.S. patent owner.

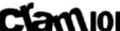

Chapter 12. Antidepressants

Reboxetine	Reboxetine is an antidepressant drug used in the treatment of clinical depression, panic disorder and ADD/ADHD, developed by Pharmacia (now Pfizer). Its mesylate (i.e. methanesulfonate) salt is sold under tradenames including Edronax, Norebox, Prolift, Solvex, Davedax or Vestra. According to a meta-analysis of 12 new-generation antidepressants, Reboxetine was 'significantly less' effective, and was less acceptable, than the other drugs in treating the acute-phase treatment of adults with unipolar major depression.
Sedation	Sedation is a medical procedure involving the administration of sedative drugs, generally to facilitate a medical procedure or diagnostic proceedure. Drugs which can be used for Sedation include propofol, etomidate, ketamine, fentanyl and midazolam.
Agonist	An Agonist is a drug that binds to a receptor of a cell and triggers a response by the cell. An Agonist often mimics the action of a naturally occurring substance. An Agonist produces an action.
Mirtazapine	Mirtazapine is a psychoactive drug of the benzazepine and tetracyclic antidepressant (TeCA) chemical classes which is used primarily as an antidepressant. It is sometimes used for its anxiolytic, hypnotic, antiemetic, orexigenic, and antihistamine or antipruritic effects. Mirtazapine was introduced by Organon International in 1994. Along with its chemical analogue and predecessor mianserin (Bolvidon, Norval, Tolvon), Mirtazapine is one of the few noradrenergic and specific serotonergic antidepressants (NaSSAs).
Antihistamine	A histamine antagonist is an agent that serves to inhibit the release or action of histamine. antihistamine can be used to describe any histamine antagonist, but it is usually reserved for the classical antihistamines that act upon the H_1 histamine receptor. antihistamines are used as treatment for allergies.

Chapter 12. Antidepressants

Trazodone	Trazodone is a psychoactive drug of the piperazine and triazolopyridine chemical classes that has antidepressant, anxiolytic, and hypnotic properties. It has been advertised that its therapeutic benefits become noticeable within the first week of administration. Trazodone has considerably less prominent anticholinergic (dry mouth, constipation, tachycardia) and sympatholytic (hypotension, sexual dysfunction consisting of erectile dysfunction and anorgasmia) side effects in comparison to most of the tricyclic antidepressants (TCAs) and tetracyclic antidepressants (TeCAs).
Insomnia	Insomnia is a symptom which can accompany several sleep, medical and psychiatric disorders, characterized by persistent difficulty falling asleep and/or staying asleep despite the opportunity. Insomnia is typically followed by functional impairment while awake. Both organic and non-organic Insomnia without other cause constitute a sleep disorder, primary Insomnia.
Norpramin	Desipramine is a tricyclic antidepressant (TCA) that inhibits the reuptake of norepinephrine and serotonin and to a lesser extent dopamine. It is sold under the brand names Norpramin and Pertofrane. It is used to treat depression, but not considered a first line treatment since the introduction of SSRI antidepressants.
Doxepin	Doxepin is a psychotropic agent with tricyclic antidepressant and anxiolytic properties, known under many brand-names such as Aponal, the original preparation by Boehringer-Mannheim, now part of the Roche group; Adapine, Deptran, Sinquan and Sinequan (Pfizer). As Doxepin hydrochloride, it is the active ingredient in cream-based preparations (Zonalon and Xepin) for the treatment of dermatological itch. Doxepin is currently investigated for the treatment of insomnia, and the proposed tradename of Doxepin for this indication is Silenor.
Mood stabilizer	A Mood stabilizer is a psychiatric medication used to treat mood disorders characterized by intense and sustained mood shifts, which is not the same as 'feeling good one minute and then bad the next.' One use is in bipolar disorder, where Mood stabilizers suppress swings between mania and depression. These drugs are also used in borderline personality disorder. Most Mood stabilizers are purely antimanic agents, meaning that they are effective at treating mania and mood cycling and shifting, but are not effective at treating depression.

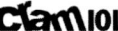

Chapter 12. Antidepressants

Nortriptyline	Nortriptyline is a second-generation tricyclic antidepressant marketed as the hydrochloride under the trade names Sensoval, Aventyl, Pamelor, Norpress, Allegron and Nortrilen. It is used in the treatment of major depression and childhood nocturnal enuresis (bedwetting). In addition, it is sometimes used for chronic illnesses such as chronic fatigue syndrome, chronic pain and migraines, and labile affect in some neurological conditions.
Abuse	Abuse is defined as:
Cocaine	Cocaine is a crystalline tropane alkaloid that is obtained from the leaves of the coca plant. The name comes from 'coca' in addition to the alkaloid suffix -ine, forming Cocaine. It is a stimulant of the central nervous system and an appetite suppressant.
Iproniazid	Iproniazid is a hydrazine drug used as an antidepressant. It acts as an irreversible and nonselective monoamine oxidase inhibitor (MAOI). Though it has been widely discontinued in most of the world, it is still used in France.
Monoamine oxidase	L-Monoamine oxidases (MAO) (EC 1.4.3.4) are a family of enzymes that catalyze the oxidation of monoamines. They are found bound to the outer membrane of mitochondria in most cell types in the body. The enzyme was originally discovered by Mary Bernheim (née Hare) in the liver and was named tyramine oxidase.
Monoamine oxidase inhibitor	Monoamine oxidase inhibitors are a class of antidepressant drugs prescribed for the treatment of depression. They are particularly effective in treating atypical depression. Because of potentially lethal dietary and drug interactions, monoamine oxidase inhibitors have historically been reserved as a last line of treatment, used only when other classes of antidepressant drugs (for example selective serotonin reuptake inhibitors and tricyclic antidepressants) have failed.
Isocarboxazid	Isocarboxazid is an irreversible and nonselective monoamine oxidase inhibitor (MAOI) of the hydrazine chemical class used as an antidepressant and anxiolytic. It is one of the few hydrazine MAOIs still in clinical use, along with phenelzine. .

Chapter 12. Antidepressants

Phenelzine	Phenelzine is an irreversible and nonselective and monoamine oxidase inhibitor (MAOI) of the hydrazine chemical class which is used as an antidepressant and anxiolytic. Along with tranylcypromine and isocarboxazid, Phenelzine is one of the few nonselective MAOIs still in widespread clinical use.
	Phenelzine and the other MAOIs are typically considered to be significantly more effective against clinical depression in comparison to more mainstream antidepressants like the selective serotonin reuptake inhibitors (SSRIs), but are usually reserved only as a last resort due to their prominent side effects and potentially hazardous food and drug interactions.
Phenethylamine	Phenethylamine is a natural monoamine alkaloid, trace amine, and psychoactive drug with stimulant effects. Studies suggest that phenylethylamine functions as a neuromodulator or neurotransmitter in the mammalian central nervous system. It is biosynthesized from the amino acid phenylalanine by enzymatic decarboxylation.
Excitotoxicity	Excitotoxicity is the pathological process by which nerve cells are damaged and killed by glutamate and similar substances. This occurs when receptors for the excitatory neurotransmitter glutamate (glutamate receptors) such as the NMDA receptor and AMPA receptor are overactivated. Excitotoxins like NMDA and kainic acid which bind to these receptors, as well as pathologically high levels of glutamate, can cause Excitotoxicity by allowing high levels of calcium ions (Ca^{2+}) to enter the cell.
Decongestant	A Decongestant or nasal Decongestant is a type of drug which is used to relieve nasal congestion.
	The vast majority of Decongestants act via enhancing norepinephrine (noradrenaline) and epinephrine (adrenaline) or adrenergic activity by stimulating the α-adrenergic receptors. This induces vasoconstriction of the blood vessels in the nose, throat, and paranasal sinuses, which results in reduced inflammation and mucus formation in these areas.
Interaction	Interaction is a kind of action that occurs as two or more objects have an effect upon one another. The idea of a two-way effect is essential in the concept of Interaction, as opposed to a one-way causal effect. A closely related term is interconnectivity, which deals with the Interactions of Interactions within systems: combinations of many simple Interactions can lead to surprising emergent phenomena.

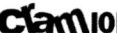

Chapter 12. Antidepressants

Bipolar disorder	Bipolar disorder or manic-depressive disorder is a psychiatric diagnosis that describes a category of mood disorders defined by the presence of one or more episodes of abnormally elevated mood clinically referred to as mania or, if milder, hypomania. Individuals who experience manic episodes also commonly experience depressive episodes or symptoms, or mixed episodes in which features of both mania and depression are present at the same time. These episodes are usually separated by periods of 'normal' mood, but in some individuals, depression and mania may rapidly alternate, known as rapid cycling.
Transdermal	Transdermal is a route of administration wherein active ingredients are delivered across the skin for systemic distribution. Examples include Transdermal patches used for medicine delivery, and Transdermal implants used for medical or aesthetic purposes. Although the skin is a large and logical target for drug delivery, its basic functions limit its utility for this purpose.
Drug interaction	A Drug interaction is a situation in which a substance affects the activity of a drug, i.e. the effects are increased or decreased, or they produce a new effect that neither produces on its own. Typically, interaction between drugs come to mind (drug-Drug interaction). However, interactions may also exist between drugs ' foods (drug-food interactions), as well as drugs ' herbs (drug-herb interactions).
Sympathomimetic drugs	Sympathomimetic drugs are substances that mimic the effects of the sympathetic nervous system, such as catecholamines, epinephrine (adrenaline), norepinephrine (noradrenaline), dopamine, etc. Such drugs are used to treat cardiac arrest, low blood pressure, or even delay premature labor, among other things. These drugs act at the postganglionic sympathetic terminal, either directly activating postsynaptic receptors, blocking breakdown and reuptake, or stimulating production and release of catecholamines.
Phenylephrine	Phenylephrine or Neo-Synephrine is an α_1-adrenergic receptor agonist used primarily as a decongestant, as an agent to dilate the pupil, and to increase blood pressure. Phenylephrine has recently been marketed as a substitute for pseudoephedrine (e.g., Pfizer's Sudafed (Original Formulation)), but there are recent claims that oral Phenylephrine may be no more effective as a decongestant than a placebo .

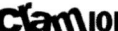

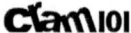

Chapter 12. Antidepressants

	Phenylephrine is used as a decongestant sold as an oral medicine, as a nasal spray, or as eye drops.
MAOIs	Monoamine oxidase inhibitors (MAOIs) are a class of powerful antidepressant drugs prescribed for the treatment of depression. They are particularly effective in treating atypical depression, and have also shown efficacy in smoking cessation. Due to potentially lethal dietary and drug interactions, MAOIs had been reserved as a last line of defense, used only when other classes of antidepressant drugs (for example selective serotonin reuptake inhibitors and tricyclic antidepressants) have failed.
Dextromethorphan	Dextromethorphan is an antitussive (cough suppressant) drug. It is one of the active ingredients in many over-the-counter cold and cough medicines, such as Robitussin, NyQuil, Dimetapp, Vicks, Coricidin, Delsym, and others, including generic labels. Dextromethorphan has also found other uses in medicine, ranging from pain relief to psychological applications.
Ephedrine	Ephedrine [pronunciation: i-Ë^fed-rÉ™n, British also Ë^ef-É™-drÉ™n] is a sympathomimetic amine commonly used as a stimulant, appetite suppressant, concentration aid, decongestant, and to treat hypotension associated with anaesthesia. Ephedrine is similar in structure to the (semi-synthetic) derivatives amphetamine and methamphetamine. Structurally, Ephedrine is a substituted amphetamine and methamphetamine analogue, Ephedrine differs from methamphetamine only by the presence of a hydroxyl (OH) group at the R^β position.
Hypertension	Hypertension is a chronic medical condition in which the blood pressure is elevated. It is also referred to as high blood pressure or shortened to HT, HTN or HPN. The word 'Hypertension', by itself, normally refers to systemic, arterial Hypertension. Hypertension can be classified as either essential (primary) or secondary.
Hypotension	Blood pressure is the force of blood pushing against the walls of the arteries as the heart pumps out blood. If it is lower than normal then it is called as low blood pressure . In physiology and medicine, Hypotension is abnormally low blood pressure.

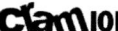

Chapter 12. Antidepressants

Phenylpropanolamine	Phenylpropanolamine (PPA; Accutrim, Dexatrim), also knwon as norephedrine and oxyamphetamine, is a psychoactive drug of the phenethylamine and amphetamine chemical classes which is used as a stimulant, decongestant, and anorectic agent. It is commonly used in prescription and over-the-counter cough and cold preparations. In veterinary medicine, it is used to control urinary incontinence in dogs under trade names Propalin and Proin.
Pseudoephedrine	Pseudoephedrine [pronunciation: soÍžoËŒEdÅ -Ä-fÄ•dˑrÄn or soÍžoËŒEdÅ -Ä•fˑÄ-drÄ"nËŒ] is a sympathomimetic drug of the phenethylamine and amphetamine chemical classes used as a nasal/sinus decongestant and stimulant or wakefulness-promoting agent. The salts Pseudoephedrine hydrochloride and Pseudoephedrine sulfate are found in many over-the-counter preparations either as single-ingredient preparations, or more commonly in combination with antihistamines, guaifenesin, dextromethorphan, paracetamol (acetaminophen), and/or NSAIDs (e.g., aspirin, ibuprofen, etc). Pseudoephedrine is a diastereomer of ephedrine.
Prolixin	Fluphenazine is a typical antipsychotic drug used for the treatment of psychoses such as schizophrenia and acute manic phases of bipolar disorder. It belongs to the piperazine class of phenothiazines and is extremely potent; more potent than haloperidol and around fifty to seventy times the potency of chlorpromazine. It is marketed under the brand name of Prolixin and Sydocate(Surge Laboratories).
Hyperthermia	Hyperthermia is an elevated body temperature due to failed thermoregulation. Hyperthermia occurs when the body produces or absorbs more heat than it can dissipate. When the elevated body temperatures are sufficiently high, hyperthermia is a medical emergency and requires immediate treatment to prevent disability or death.
Pethidine	Pethidine is a fast-acting opioid analgesic drug. In the United States and Canada, it is more commonly known as meperidine or by its brand name Demerol.
Serotonin syndrome	Serotonin syndrome is a potentially life-threatening adverse drug reaction that may occur following therapeutic drug use, inadvertent interactions between drugs, overdose of particular drugs, or the recreational use of certain drugs. Serotonin syndrome is not an idiosyncratic drug reaction; it is a predictable consequence of excess serotonergic activity at central nervous system (CNS) and peripheral serotonin receptors. For this reason, some experts strongly prefer the terms serotonin toxicity or serotonin toxidrome because these more accurately reflect the fact that it is a form of poisoning.

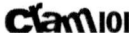

Chapter 12. Antidepressants

Tramadol	Tramadol is a centrally acting analgesic, used for treating moderate to severe pain.
	Tramadol was developed by the German pharmaceutical company Grünenthal GmbH in the late 1970s.
	Tramadol possesses agonist actions at the μ-opioid receptor and affects reuptake at the noradrenergic and serotonergic systems.
Desipramine	Desipramine is a tricyclic antidepressant (TCA) that inhibits the reuptake of norepinephrine and serotonin and to a lesser extent dopamine. It is sold under the brand names Norpramin and Pertofrane. It is used to treat depression, but not considered a first line treatment since the introduction of SSRI antidepressants.
Adrenergic receptors	The Adrenergic receptors are a class of G protein-coupled receptors that are targets of the catecholamines, especially noradrenaline (norepinephrine) and adrenaline (epinephrine). Although dopamine is a catecholamine, its receptors are in a different category.
	Many cells possess these receptors, and the binding of an agonist will generally cause a sympathetic response (e.g. the fight-or-flight response). For instance, the heart rate will increase and the pupils will dilate, energy will be mobilized, and blood flow diverted from other non-essential organs to skeletal muscle.
Atypical antipsychotics	The Atypical antipsychotics are a group of antipsychotic drugs used to treat psychiatric conditions. Some Atypical antipsychotics are FDA approved for use in the treatment of schizophrenia. Some carry FDA approved indications for acute mania, bipolar mania, psychotic agitation, bipolar maintenance, and other indications.
Pharmacokinetics	Pharmacokinetics is a branch of pharmacology dedicated to the determination of the fate of substances administered externally to a living organism. In practice, this discipline is applied mainly to drug substances, though in principle it concerns itself with all manner of compounds ingested or otherwise delivered externally to an organism, such as nutrients, metabolites, hormones, toxins, etc.
	pharmacokinetics is often studied in conjunction with pharmacodynamics.

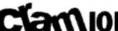

Chapter 12. Antidepressants

Benadryl	Benadryl is a brand name allergy medicine marketed over-the-counter by Johnson ' Johnson subsidiary McNeil Consumer Healthcare. Prior to 2007, Benadryl was marketed by Pfizer Consumer Healthcare. Benadryl is used as an antihistamine for the temporary relief of seasonal and perennial allergy symptoms.
Atorvastatin	Atorvastatin is a member of the drug class known as statins, used for lowering blood cholesterol. It also stabilizes plaque and prevents strokes through anti-inflammatory and other mechanisms.
	Atorvastatin inhibits HMG-CoA reductase, the rate-determining enzyme located in hepatic tissue that produces mevalonate, a small molecule used in the synthesis of cholesterol and other mevalonate derivatives. This lowers the amount of cholesterol produced which in turn lowers the total amount of LDL cholesterol. Atorvastatin was first synthesized in 1985 by Bruce Roth while working at Parke-Davis Warner-Lambert Company (now Pfizer).
Simvastatin	Simvastatin is a hypolipidemic drug belonging to the class of pharmaceuticals called 'statins'. It is used to control hypercholesterolemia (elevated cholesterol levels) and to prevent cardiovascular disease. Simvastatin is a synthetic derivate of a fermentation product of Aspergillus terreus.
Triazolam	Triazolam is a benzodiazepine derivative drug. It possesses pharmacological properties similar to that of other benzodiazepines, but it is generally only used as a sedative to treat insomnia. In addition to the hypnotic properties Triazolam possesses, amnesic, anxiolytic, sedative, anticonvulsant and muscle relaxant properties are also present.
Trifluoperazine	Trifluoperazine is a typical antipsychotic drug of the phenothiazine group.
	Trifluoperazine has central antiadrenergic, antidopaminergic, and minimal anticholinergic effects. It is believed to work by blockading dopamine D_1 and D_2 receptors in the mesocortical and mesolimbic pathways, relieving or minimizing such symptoms of schizophrenia as hallucinations, delusions, and disorganized thought and speech.
Antibiotic	In common usage, an Antibiotic is a substance or compound that kills, or inhibits the growth of, bacteria. Antibiotics belong to the broader group of antimicrobial compounds, used to treat infections caused by microorganisms, including fungi and protozoa.

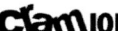

Chapter 12. Antidepressants

	The term 'Antibiotic' was coined by Selman Waksman in 1942 to describe any substance produced by a microorganism that is antagonistic to the growth of other microorganisms in high dilution.
Erythromycin	Erythromycin is a macrolide antibiotic that has an antimicrobial spectrum similar to or slightly wider than that of penicillin, and is often used for people who have an allergy to penicillins. For respiratory tract infections, it has better coverage of atypical organisms, including mycoplasma and Legionellosis. It was first marketed by Eli Lilly and Company, and it is today commonly known as EES (Erythromycin ethylsuccinate, an ester prodrug that is commonly administered).
Fluvastatin	Fluvastatin is a member of the drug class of statins, used to treat hypercholesterolemia and to prevent cardiovascular disease. It has also been shown to exhibit antiviral activity against Hepatitis C.
Macrolide	The macrolides are a group of drugs (typically antibiotics) whose activity stems from the presence of a macrolide ring, a large macrocyclic lactone ring to which one or more deoxy sugars, usually cladinose and desosamine, may be attached. The lactone rings are usually 14, 15 or 16-membered. macrolides belong to the polyketide class of natural products. · Azithromycin (Zithromax, Zitromax, Sumamed, Azitrox) - Unique, does not inhibit CYP3A4 · Clarithromycin (Biaxin, Fromilid, Klacid, Klabax, Lekoklar) · Dirithromycin (Dynabac) · Erythromycin · Roxithromycin (Rulid, Surlid, Roxid) · Telithromycin · Carbomycin A · Josamycin

Chapter 12. Antidepressants

· Kitasamycin

· Midecamicine/midecamicine acetate

· Oleandomycin

· Spiramycin

· Troleandomycin

· Tylosin/tylocine (Tylan)

Ketolides are a new class of antibiotics that are structurally related to the macrolides.

Pravastatin	Pravastatin is a member of the drug class of statins, used for lowering cholesterol and preventing cardiovascular disease. Initially known as CS-514, it was originally identified in a bacterium called Nocardia autotrophica by researchers of the Sankyo Pharma Inc.. It is presently being marketed outside Japan by the pharmaceutical company Bristol-Myers Squibb.
Triglycerides	(more properly known as , TAG or triacylglyceride) is a glyceride in which the glycerol is esterified with three fatty acids. It is the main constituent of vegetable oil and animal fats.
	Triglycerides are formed from a single molecule of glycerol, combined with three fatty acids on each of the OH groups, and make up most of fats digested by humans.
Estazolam	Estazolam is a drug which is a benzodiazepine derivative. It possesses anxiolytic, anticonvulsant, sedative and skeletal muscle relaxant properties. Estazolam is an intermediate-acting oral benzodiazepine.
Estradiol	Estradiol (also oEstradiol) is a sex hormone. Estradiol is the predominant sex hormone present in females; however, it is present in males, albeit at lower levels, as well. It represents the major estrogen in humans.

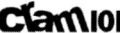

Chapter 12. Antidepressants

Estrogen receptor	Estrogen receptor refers to a group of receptors that are activated by the hormone 17β-estradiol (estrogen). Two types of estrogen receptor exist: Estrogen receptor, which is a member of the nuclear hormone family of intracellular receptors, and the estrogen G protein-coupled receptor GPR30 (GPER), which is a G protein-coupled receptor.
Amyloid	Amyloids are insoluble fibrous protein aggregates sharing specific structural traits. Abnormal accumulation of amyloid in organs may lead to amyloidosis, and may play a role in various neurodegenerative diseases. The name amyloid comes from the early mistaken identification of the substance as starch, based on crude iodine-staining techniques.
Brain-derived neurotrophic factor	Brain-derived neurotrophic factor is a protein that, in humans, is encoded by the Brain derived neurotrophic factor gene. Brain derived neurotrophic factor is a member of the 'neurotrophin' family of growth factors, which are related to the canonical 'Nerve Growth Factor', NGF. Neurotrophic factors are found in the brain and the periphery.
Glutamate receptors	Glutamate receptors are synaptic receptors located primarily on the membranes of neuronal cells. Glutamate is one of the 20 amino acids used to assemble proteins and as a result is abundant in many areas of the body, but it also functions as a neurotransmitter and is particularly abundant in the nervous system. Glutamate receptors are responsible for the glutamate-mediated post-synaptic excitation of neural cells, and are important for neural communication, memory formation, learning, and regulation.
Progesterone	Progesterone also known as P4 (pregn-4-ene-3,20-dione) is a C-21 steroid hormone involved in the female menstrual cycle, pregnancy (supports gestation) and embryogenesis of humans and other species. Progesterone belongs to a class of hormones called progestogens, and is the major naturally occurring human progestogen. Progesterone is commonly manufactured from the yam family, Dioscorea.
Menstrual cycle	The menstrual cycle is the scientific term for the physiological changes that can occur in fertile female humans and apes. Overt menstruation (where there is blood flow from the uterus through the vagina) occurs in humans and some animals such as chimpanzees. Females of other species of placental mammal undergo estrous cycles, in which the endometrium is completely reabsorbed by the animal (covert menstruation) at the end of its reproductive cycle.

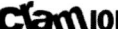

Chapter 12. Antidepressants

Premenstrual syndrome	Premenstrual syndrome is a collection of physical and emotional symptoms related to a woman's menstrual cycle. While most women of child-bearing age (up to 85%) report having experienced physical symptoms related to normal ovulatory function, such as bloating or breast tenderness, medical definitions of PMS are limited to a consistent pattern of emotional and physical symptoms occurring only during the luteal phase of the menstrual cycle that are of 'sufficient severity to interfere with some aspects of life'. In particular, emotional symptoms must be present consistently to diagnose PMS. The specific emotional and physical symptoms attributable to PMS vary from woman to woman, but each individual woman's pattern of symptoms is predictable, occurs consistently during the fourteen days prior to menses, and vanishes either shortly before or shortly after the start of menstrual flow.
Psychosis	Psychosis means abnormal condition of the mind, and is a generic psychiatric term for a mental state often described as involving a 'loss of contact with reality'. People suffering from Psychosis are said to be psychotic.

People experiencing Psychosis may report hallucinations or delusional beliefs, and may exhibit personality changes and thought disorder. |
| Clonidine | clonidine is a medication used to treat several medical conditions. It is a direct-acting α2 adrenergic agonist.

It has been prescribed historically as an antihypertensive agent. |
| Folinic acid | Folinic acid or leucovorin (USAN), generally administered as calcium or sodium folinate (or leucovorin calcium/sodium), is an adjuvant used in cancer chemotherapy involving the drug methotrexate. It is also used in synergistic combination with the chemotherapy agent 5-fluorouracil.

LevoFolinic acid and its salts are the enantiopure drugs. |
| Folic acid | Folic acid and folate (the naturally occurring form), as well as pteroyl-L-glutamic acid and pteroyl-L-glutamate, are forms of the water-soluble vitamin B_9. Folic acid is itself not biologically active, but its biological importance is due to tetrahydrofolate and other derivatives after its conversion to dihydroFolic acid in the liver. |

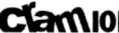

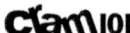

Chapter 12. Antidepressants

	Vitamin B_9 (Folic acid and folate inclusive) is essential to numerous bodily functions ranging from nucleotide biosynthesis to the remethylation of homocysteine.
Thyroid	The Thyroid is one of the largest endocrine glands in the body. This gland is found in the neck, inferior to (below) the Thyroid cartilage (also known as the Adam's apple) and at approximately the same level as the cricoid cartilage. The Thyroid controls how quickly the body uses energy, makes proteins, and controls how sensitive the body should be to other hormones.
Thyroid hormone	The Thyroid hormones, thyroxine (T_4) and triiodothyronine (T_3), are tyrosine-based hormones produced by the thyroid gland primarily responsible for regulation of metabolism. An important component in the synthesis of Thyroid hormones is iodine. The major form of Thyroid hormone in the blood is thyroxine (T_4), which has a longer half life than T_3.
Lithium	Lithium is a soft, silver-white metal that belongs to the alkali metal group of chemical elements. It is represented by the symbol Li, and it has the atomic number three. Under standard conditions it is the lightest metal and the least dense solid element.
Electroconvulsive therapy	Electroconvulsive therapy is a psychiatric treatment in which seizures are electrically induced in anesthetized patients for therapeutic effect. Its mode of action is unknown. Today, electroconvulsive therapy is most often recommended for use as a treatment for severe depression which has not responded to other treatment, and is also used in the treatment of mania and catatonia.
Vagus nerve	The vagus nerve is the tenth of twelve (excluding CN0) paired cranial nerves. Upon leaving the medulla between the olivary nucleus and the inferior cerebellar peduncle, it extends through the jugular foramen, then passing into the carotid sheath between the internal carotid artery and the internal jugular vein down below the head, to the neck, chest and abdomen, where it contributes to the innervation of the viscera. Besides output to the various organs in the body, the vagus nerve conveys sensory information about the state of the body's organs to the central nervous system. 80-90% of the nerve fibers in the vagus nerve are afferent (sensory) nerves communicating the state of the viscera to the brain.
Pharmacy	Pharmacy is the health profession that links the health sciences with the chemical sciences and it is charged with ensuring the safe and effective use of pharmaceutical drugs.

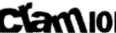

Chapter 12. Antidepressants

The scope of pharmacy practice includes more traditional roles such as compounding and dispensing medications, and it also includes more modern services related to health care, including clinical services, reviewing medications for safety and efficacy, and providing drug information. Pharmacists, therefore, are the experts on drug therapy and are the primary health professionals who optimize medication use to provide patients with positive health outcomes.

Algorithm

In mathematics, computer science, and related subjects, an Algorithm is an effective method for solving a problem using a finite sequence of instructions. Algorithms are used for calculation, data processing, and many other fields.

Each Algorithm is a list of well-defined instructions for completing a task.

Buspirone

Buspirone is a psychoactive drug and pharmaceutical medication of the piperazine and azapirone chemical classes. It is used primarily as an anxiolytic, but also to a lesser extent as an antidepressant. Bristol-Myers Squibb (BMS) gained Food and Drug Administration (FDA) approval for Buspirone in 1986, and it went generic in 2001.

Gepirone

Gepirone is a psychoactive drug and research chemical of the piperazine and azapirone chemical classes. It is currently under clinical development in an extended release form as an anxiolytic and antidepressant agent. Pharmacologically, Gepirone acts as a selective 5-HT_{1A} receptor partial agonist.

Pindolol

Pindolol is a beta blocker.

Pindolol is a nonselective beta blocker with partial beta-adrenergic receptor agonist activity. It possesses ISA (Intrinsic Sympathomimetic Activity). This means that Pindolol particularly in high doses exerts effects like epinephrine or isoprenaline (increased pulse rate, increased blood pressure, bronchodilation), but these effects are limited. Pindolol also shows membrane stabilizing effects like quinidine, possibly accounting for its antiarrhythmic effects.

Standard

A technical standard is an established norm or requirement. It is usually a formal document that establishes uniform engineering or technical criteria, methods, processes and practices. In contrast, a custom, convention, company product, corporate standard, etc which becomes generally accepted and dominant is often called a de facto standard.

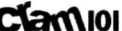

Chapter 12. Antidepressants

Modafinil	Modafinil is an analeptic drug manufactured by Cephalon, and is approved by the U.S. Food and Drug Administration (FDA) for the treatment of narcolepsy, shift work sleep disorder, and excessive daytime sleepiness associated with obstructive sleep apnea.
	Modafinil, like other stimulants, increases the release of monoamines, specifically the catecholamines norepinephrine and dopamine, from the synaptic terminals. However, Modafinil also elevates hypothalamic histamine levels, leading some researchers to consider Modafinil a 'wakefulness promoting agent' rather than a classic amphetamine-like stimulant (as evidenced by the difference in c-Fos distribution caused by Modafinil as compared to amphetamine).
Rheumatology	Rheumatology is a sub-specialty in internal medicine and pediatrics, devoted to diagnosis and therapy of conditions and diseases affecting joints, muscles, and bones. Clinicians who specialize in rheumatology are called rheumatologists. Rheumatologists deal mainly with clinical problems involving joints, soft tissues, certain autoimmune diseases, vasculitis, and heritable connective tissue disorders.
Amibegron	Amibegron (SR-58,611A) is a drug developed by Sanofi-Aventis which acts as a selective agonist for the β3 adrenergic receptor. It is the first orally active β3 agonist developed that is capable of entering the Central Nervous System, and has antidepressant and anxiolytic effects. On July 31, 2008, Sanofi-Aventis announced that it has decided to discontinue development of Amibegron.
Fibromyalgia	Fibromyalgia is also referred to as FM or FMS. Fibromyalgia is characterized by chronic widespread pain and allodynia, a heightened and painful response to pressure.
Melanocytes	Melanocytes) are melanin-producing cells located in the bottom layer (the stratum basale) of the skin's epidermis, the middle layer of the eye (the uvea), the inner ear, meninges, bones, and heart. Melanin is a pigment which is responsible for the color of skin, among other things.
Nemifitide	Nemifitide is an experimental, unapproved drug which has been studied for efficacy as an antidepressant in animal testing. Chemically unrelated to existing approved antidepressants, Nemifitide has a molecular structure similar to melanocyte-inhibiting factor.page 303

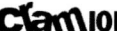

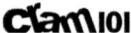
Nemifitide has been shown to exhibit activity as an antagonist at the 5-HT$_{2A}$ serotonin receptor subtype, because it prevents the development of fever ordinarily induced by administration of 2,5-Dimethoxy-4-iodoamphetamine. It is believed that the compound's effectiveness as an antidepressant is mediated, at least in part, via serotonergic mechanisms.[page 307]

1. [a] [b] [c] Overstreet DH, Hlavka J, Feighner JP, Nicolau G, Freed JS (September 2004).

Opiate

In medicine, the term Opiate describes any of the narcotic opioid alkaloids found as natural products in the opium poppy plant, as well as many semisynthetic chemical derivatives of such alkaloids.

Opiates are so named because they are constituents or derivatives of constituents found in opium, which is processed from the latex sap of the opium poppy, Papaver somniferum. The major biologically active Opiates found in opium are morphine, codeine, thebaine, and papaverine.

Saredutant

Saredutant is a drug which acts as a NK$_2$ receptor antagonist. It was under development by Sanofi-Aventis as a novel antidepressant and anxiolytic and made it to phase III clinical trials. However, in May of 2009, Sanofi-Aventis published its quarterly results and announced the cessation of 14 research/development projects, among which was Saredutant for the treatment of major depressive disorder..

Anticonvulsant

The anticonvulsants are a diverse group of pharmaceuticals used in the treatment of epileptic seizures. anticonvulsants are also increasingly being used in the treatment of bipolar disorder, since many seem to act as mood stabilizers. The goal of an anticonvulsant is to suppress the rapid and excessive firing of neurons that start a seizure.

Pamelor

Nortriptyline is a second-generation tricyclic antidepressant marketed as the hydrochloride under the trade names Sensoval, Aventyl, Pamelor, Norpress, Allegron and Nortrilen. It is used in the treatment of major depression and childhood nocturnal enuresis (bedwetting). In addition, it is sometimes used for chronic illnesses such as chronic fatigue syndrome, chronic pain and migraines, and labile affect in some neurological conditions.

Valproic acid

Valproic acid (VPA) is a chemical compound that has found clinical use as an anticonvulsant and mood-stabilizing drug, primarily in the treatment of epilepsy, bipolar disorder, and less commonly major depression. It is also used to treat migraine headaches and schizophrenia. It is marketed under the brand names Depakote, Depakote ER, Depakene, Depacon, Stavzor.

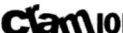

Chapter 12. Antidepressants

Carbamazepine	Carbamazepine (CBZ) is an anticonvulsant and mood stabilizing drug used primarily in the treatment of epilepsy and bipolar disorder, as well as trigeminal neuralgia. It is also used off-label for a variety of indications, including attention-deficit hyperactivity disorder (ADHD), schizophrenia, phantom limb syndrome, paroxysmal extreme pain disorder, and post-traumatic stress disorder. Carbamazepine was discovered by chemist Walter Schindler at J.R. Geigy AG (now part of Novartis) in Basel, Switzerland, in 1953.
Valium	Diazepam , first marketed as Valium by Hoffmann-La Roche, is a benzodiazepine derivative drug. It is commonly used for treating anxiety, insomnia, seizures, muscle spasms, restless legs syndrome, alcohol withdrawal, benzodiazepine withdrawal, and Ménière's disease. It may also be used before certain medical procedures to reduce tension and anxiety, and in some surgical procedures to induce amnesia.
Bone marrow	Bone marrow is the flexible tissue found in the hollow interior of bones. In adults, marrow in large bones produces new blood cells. It constitutes 4% of total body weight, i.e. approximately 2.6 kg (5.7 lbs).
Oxcarbazepine	Oxcarbazepine is an anticonvulsant and mood stabilizing drug, used primarily in the treatment of epilepsy. It is also used to treat anxiety and mood disorders, and benign motor tics. Oxcarbazepine is marketed as Trileptal by Novartis and in Egypt is marketed also as Oxaleptal 600mg by Mash Premiere and available in some countries as a generic drug.
First-line treatment	A First-line treatment or first-line therapy is a medical therapy recommended for the initial treatment of a disease, sign or symptom, usually on the basis of empirical evidence for its efficacy. This evidence, often based on scientific research studies, of which the randomized controlled trial is the gold standard, typically suggests the recommended therapy is most likely to have an effect for the given condition. Alternative treatment options, including switching to another treatment, or augmenting the First-line treatment with another treatment, may be recommended if the first-line therapy does not ease the symptoms, or produces intolerable side effects.
Lamotrigine	Lamotrigine by GlaxoSmithKline, called Lamictin in South Africa, ×œ×žž×•××''×™×Ÿ in Israel, and ë ¼ë¯¹ìí in South Korea and also Lamitor) is an anticonvulsant drug used in the treatment of epilepsy and bipolar disorder. For epilepsy it is used to treat partial seizures, primary and secondary tonic-clonic seizures, and seizures associated with Lennox-Gastaut syndrome. Lamotrigine also acts as a mood stabilizer.

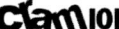

Chapter 12. Antidepressants

Rashes	A rash is a change of the skin which affects its color, appearance or texture. A rash may be localized in one part of the body, or affect all the skin. Rashes may cause the skin to change color, itch, become warm, bumpy, dry, cracked or blistered, swell and may be painful.
Toxic epidermal necrolysis	Toxic epidermal necrolysis is a rare, life-threatening dermatological condition that is usually induced by a reaction to medications. It is characterized by the detachment of the top layer of skin (the epidermis) from the lower layers of the skin (the dermis) all over the body.
	There is broad agreement in medical literature that Toxic epidermal necrolysis can be considered a more severe form of Stevens-Johnson syndrome, and debate whether it falls on a spectrum of disease that includes erythema multiforme.
Topiramate	Topiramate is an anticonvulsant drug produced by Ortho-McNeil Neurologics and Noramco, Inc., both being divisions of Johnson ' Johnson. It was discovered in 1979 by Bruce E. Maryanoff and Joseph F. Gardocki during their research work at McNeil Pharmaceutical. Generic versions are available in Canada and were FDA approved in September 2006. Mylan Pharmaceuticals was recently granted final approval for generic Topiramate 25, 100, and 200 mg tablets and sprinkle capsules by the FDA for sale in the US. 50 mg tablets were granted tentative approval.
Gabapentin	Gabapentin is a GABA analogue. It was originally developed for the treatment of epilepsy, and currently, Gabapentin is widely used to relieve pain, especially neuropathic pain.
	Gabapentin was initially synthesized to mimic the chemical structure of the neurotransmitter gamma-aminobutyric acid (GABA), but is not believed to act on the same brain receptors.
Pregabalin	Pregabalin is an anticonvulsant drug used for neuropathic pain and as an adjunct therapy for partial seizures with or without secondary generalization in adults. It has also been found effective for generalized anxiety disorder and is approved for this use in the European Union. It was designed as a more potent successor to gabapentin.
Probability	Probability is a way of expressing knowledge or belief that an event will occur or has occurred. The concept has an exact mathematical meaning in probability theory, which is used extensively in such areas of study as mathematics, statistics, finance, gambling, science, artificial intelligence/machine learning and philosophy to draw conclusions about the likelihood of potential events and the underlying mechanics of complex systems.

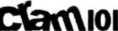

Chapter 12. Antidepressants

Substance abuse	Although the term substance can refer to any physical matter, Substance abuse has come to refer to the overindulgence in and dependence of a drug or other chemical leading to effects that are detrimental to the individual's physical and mental health, or the welfare of others. Source: A Public Health Approach to Drug Control in Canada, Health Officers Council of British Columbia, 2005
	The disorder is characterized by a pattern of continued pathological use of a medication, non-medically indicated drug or toxin, that results in repeated adverse social consequences related to drug use, such as failure to meet work, family, or school obligations, interpersonal conflicts, or legal problems. There are on-going debates as to the exact distinctions between Substance abuse and substance dependence, but current practice standard distinguishes between the two by defining substance dependence in terms of physiological and behavioral symptoms of substance use, and Substance abuse in terms of the social consequences of substance use.
Zonisamide	Zonisamide is a sulfonamide anticonvulsant approved for use as an adjunctive therapy in adults with partial-onset seizures for adults; infantile spasm, mixed seizure types of Lennox-Gastaut syndrome, myoclonic, and generalized tonic clonic seizure.
	Zonisamide was discovered by Uno and colleagues in 1972 and launched by Dainippon Sumitomo Pharma) in 1989 as Excegran in Japan. It was marketed by Élan in the United States starting in 2000 as Zonegran, before Élan transferred their interests in Zonisamide to Eisai in 2004. Eisai also markets Zonegran in Asia (China, Taiwan, and fourteen others) and Europe .
Somatic	The term somatic means 'of the body'. It is often used in biology to refer to the cells of the body in contrast to the cells in the germline which give rise to the gametes (eggs or sperm). These somatic cells are diploid containing two copies of each chromosome, whereas the germ cells are haploid as they only contain one copy of each chromosome.
Amantadine	Amantadine is the organic compound known formally as 1-aminoadamantane. The molecule consists of adamantane backbone that is substituted at one of the four methyne positions with an amino group. This compound is sold under the name 'Symmetrel' for use both as an antiviral and an antiparkinsonian drug.
Ketamine	Ketamine is a drug used in human and veterinary medicine developed by Parke-Davis (today a part of Pfizer) in 1962. Its hydrochloride salt is sold as Ketanest, Ketaset, and Ketalar. Pharmacologically, Ketamine is classified as an NMDA receptor antagonist.

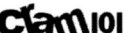

Chapter 12. Antidepressants

Memantine	Memantine is the first in a novel class of Alzheimer's disease medications acting on the glutamatergic system by blocking NMDA glutamate receptors. Memantine is marketed under the brands Axura and Akatinol by Merz, Namenda by Forest, Ebixa and Abixa by Lundbeck and Memox by Unipharm. Although Memantine is approved for treatment of moderate to severe Alzheimer's disease, its usage has been recommended against by the UK's National Institute for Clinical Excellence, on the grounds that its high cost outweighs the benefits of treatment in most patients.
Phencyclidine	Phencyclidine, commonly initialized as PCP, is a recreational dissociative drug. Formerly used as an anesthetic agent, PCP exhibits both hallucinogenic and neurotoxic effects.
Calcium	Calcium is the chemical element with the symbol Ca and atomic number 20. It has an atomic mass of 40.078 amu. Calcium is a soft gray alkaline earth metal, and is the fifth most abundant element by mass in the Earth's crust. Calcium is also the fifth most abundant dissolved ion in seawater by both molarity and mass, after sodium, chloride, magnesium, and sulfate.
Calcium channel	A Calcium channel is an ion channel which displays selective permeabiltiy to calcium ions. It is sometimes synonymous as voltage-dependent Calcium channel, although there are also ligand-gated Calcium channels. The following tables explain gating, gene, location and function of different types of Calcium channels, both voltage and ligand-gated. · the receptor-operated Calcium channels (in vasoconstriction) · P2X receptor Calcium channel blockers are used to treat hypertension.
Calcium channel blockers	calcium channel blockers are a class of drugs and natural substances that disrupt the calcium (Ca^{2+}) conduction of calcium channels. It has effects on many excitable cells of the body, such as cardiac muscle, i.e. heart, smooth muscles of blood vessels, or neurons. Drugs used to target neurons are used as antiepileptics and are not covered in this article.

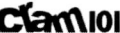

Chapter 12. Antidepressants

Channel blocker	A channel blocker is a type of drug which binds inside the pore of a specific type of ion channel and blocks the flow of ions through it, resulting in an alteration of the electrochemical gradient of the cell membrane of neurons and therefore a change in neurotransmission.
Venlafaxine	Venlafaxine is an arylalkanolamine serotonin-norepinephrine reuptake inhibitor (SNRI). First introduced by Wyeth in 1993, it is licensed for the treatment of major depressive disorder (MDD), as an anxiolytic, and comorbid indications. In 2007, Venlafaxine was the sixth most commonly prescribed antidepressant on the U.S. retail market, with 17.2 million prescriptions.
Action of drugs	The action of drugs on the human body is called pharmacodynamics, and what the body does with the drug is called pharmacokinetics. The drugs that enter the human tend to stimulate certain receptors, ion channels, act on enzymes or transporter proteins. As a result, they cause the human body to react in a specific way.
Inositol	Inositol or cyclohexane-1,2,3,4,5,6-hexol is a chemical compound with formula $C_6H_{12}O_6$ or (-CHOH-)$_6$, a six-fold alcohol (polyol) of cyclohexane. It exists in nine possible stereoisomers, of which the most prominent form, widely occuring in nature, is cis-1,2,3,5-trans-4,6-cyclohexanehexol, or myo-Inositol. Other naturally occurring isomers (though in minimal quantities) are scyllo-, muco-, D-chiro-, and neo-Inositol.
Periaqueductal gray	Periaqueductal gray is the gray matter located around the cerebral aqueduct within the tegmentum of the midbrain. It plays a role in the descending modulation of pain and in defensive behaviour. The ascending pain and temperature fibers of the spinothalamic tract also send information to the PAG via the spinomesencephalic tract .
Autism	Autism is a disorder of neural development characterized by impaired social interaction and communication, and by restricted and repetitive behavior. These signs all begin before a child is three years old. Autism affects information processing in the brain by altering how nerve cells and their synapses connect and organize; how this occurs is not well understood.
Zaleplon	Zaleplon is a sedative/hypnotic, mainly used for insomnia. It is a nonbenzodiazepine hypnotic from the pyrazolopyrimidine class. In terms of adverse effects Zaleplon appears to offer little improvement compared to both benzodiazepines and other non-benzodiazepine Z-drugs.
Ziprasidone	Ziprasidone was the fifth atypical antipsychotic to gain FDA approval (February 2001). In the United States, Ziprasidone is Food and Drug Administration (FDA) approved for the treatment of schizophrenia, and the intramuscular injection form of Ziprasidone is approved for acute agitation in schizophrenic patients. Ziprasidone has also received approval for acute treatment of mania and mixed states associated with bipolar disorder.

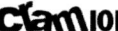

Chapter 12. Antidepressants

Quazepam	Quazepam is a drug which is a benzodiazepine derivative. Quazepam is indicated for the treatment of insomnia including sleep induction and sleep maintenance. Quazepam induces impairment of motor function and has hypnotic and anticonvulsant properties with less overdose potential than other benzodiazepines.
Dopamine agonist	A Dopamine agonist is a compound that activates dopamine receptors in the absence of the dopamine ligand. Dopamine agonists activate signaling pathways through the dopamine receptor and trimeric G-proteins, ultimately leading to changes in gene transcription.
Pramipexole	Pramipexole is a medication indicated for treating Parkinson's disease and restless legs syndrome (RLS). It is also sometimes used off-label as a treatment for cluster headache and to counteract the problems with sexual dysfunction experienced by some users of the selective serotonin reuptake inhibitor (SSRI) antidepressants. Pramipexole has shown robust effects on pilot studies in a placebo-controlled proof of concept study in bipolar disorder.
Quinidine	quinidine is a pharmaceutical agent that acts as a class I antiarrhythmic agent (Ia) in the heart. It is a stereoisomer of quinine, originally derived from the bark of the cinchona tree. Like all other class I antiarrhythmic agents, quinidine primarily works by blocking the fast inward sodium current (I_{Na}).
Ropinirole	Ropinirole is a non-ergoline dopamine agonist. It is manufactured by GlaxoSmithKline (GSK) and Sun Pharmaceutical. It is used in the treatment of Parkinson's disease.
Arteries	Arteries are blood vessels that carry blood away from the heart. All Arteries, with the exception of the pulmonary and umbilical Arteries, carry oxygenated blood. The circulatory system is extremely important for sustaining life.
Coronary arteries	Coronary circulation is the circulation of blood in the blood vessels of the heart muscle. Although blood fills the chambers of the heart, the muscle tissue of the heart (the myocardium) is so thick that it requires coronary blood vessels to deliver blood deep into it. The vessels that deliver oxygen-rich blood to the myocardium are known as Coronary arteries.

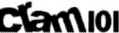

Chapter 12. Antidepressants

Cortisol	Cortisol is a corticosteroid hormone or glucocorticoid produced by the adrenal cortex, that is part of the adrenal gland (in the zona fasciculata and the zona reticularis of the adrenal cortex). It is usually referred to as the 'stress hormone' as it is involved in response to stress and anxiety, controlled by CRH. It increases blood pressure and blood sugar, and reduces immune responses. Various synthetic forms of Cortisol are used to treat a variety of different illnesses.
Atherosclerosis	Atherosclerosis is the condition in which an artery wall thickens as the result of a build-up of fatty materials such as cholesterol. It is a syndrome affecting arterial blood vessels, a chronic inflammatory response in the walls of arteries, in large part due to the accumulation of macrophage white blood cells and promoted by Low-density lipoproteins (plasma proteins that carry cholesterol and triglycerides) without adequate removal of fats and cholesterol from the macrophages by functional high density lipoproteins (HDL). It is commonly referred to as a hardening or furring of the arteries.
Autonomic nervous system	The Autonomic nervous system is the part of the peripheral nervous system that acts as a control system functioning largely below the level of consciousness, and controls visceral functions. The Autonomic nervous system affects heart rate, digestion, respiration rate, salivation, perspiration, diameter of the pupils, micturition (urination), and sexual arousal. Whereas most of its actions are involuntary, some, such as breathing, work in tandem with the conscious mind.
Ischemia	In medicine, Ischemia is a restriction in blood supply, generally due to factors in the blood vessels, with resultant damage or dysfunction of tissue. It may also be spelled ischaemia or ischæmia. Rather than hypoxia , Ischemia is an absolute or relative shortage of the blood supply to an organ, i.e. a shortage of oxygen, glucose and other blood-borne fuels.
Nervous system	The Nervous system is an organ system containing a network of specialized cells called neurons that coordinate the actions of an animal and transmit signals between different parts of its body. In most animals the Nervous system consists of two parts, central and peripheral. The central Nervous system contains the brain and spinal cord.
Flumazenil	Flumazenil is a benzodiazepine antagonist. It was introduced in 1987 by Hoffmann-La Roche under the trade name Anexate. Flumazenil is of benefit in patients who become excessively drowsy after benzodiazepines are used for either diagnostic or therapeutic procedures.

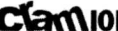
275

Go to **Cram101.com** for Interactive Practice Exams for this book or virtually any of your books.
And, **NEVER** highlight a book again!

Chapter 12. Antidepressants

Anxiolytic	An Anxiolytic (antipanic or antianxiety agent) is a drug prescribed for the treatment of symptoms of anxiety. Some Anxiolytics have been shown to be useful in the treatment of anxiety disorders, as have antidepressants such as the class of selective serotonin reuptake inhibitors (SSRIs). Though not Anxiolytics, beta-receptor blockers such as propranolol and oxprenolol can be used to combat the somatic symptoms of anxiety.
Panic disorder	Panic disorder is an anxiety disorder characterized by recurring severe panic attacks. It may also include significant behavioral change lasting at least a month and of ongoing worry about the implications or concern about having other attacks. The latter are called anticipatory attacks (DSM-IVR).
Atrophy	Atrophy is the partial or complete wasting away of a part of the body. Causes of Atrophy include poor nourishment, poor circulation, loss of hormonal support, loss of nerve supply to the target organ, disuse or lack of exercise or disease intrinsic to the tissue itself. Hormonal and nerve inputs that maintain an organ or body part are referred to as trophic [noun] in medical practice.
Glucocorticoid	Glucocorticoids (GC) are a class of steroid hormones that bind to the Glucocorticoid receptor (GR), which is present in almost every vertebrate animal cell. The name Glucocorticoid derives from their role in the regulation of the metabolism of glucose, their synthesis in the adrenal cortex, and their steroidal structure .

GCs are part of the feedback mechanism in the immune system that turns immune activity (inflammation) down. |
| Ligand | In coordination chemistry, a ligand is an ion or molecule that binds to a central metal atom to form a coordination complex. The bonding between metal and ligand generally involves formal donation of one or more of the ligand's electron pairs. The nature of metal-ligand bonding can range from covalent to ionic. |
| Generalized anxiety disorder | Generalized anxiety disorder is an anxiety disorder that is characterized by excessive, uncontrollable and often irrational worry about everyday things that is disproportionate to the actual source of worry. This excessive worry often interferes with daily functioning, as individuals suffering Generalized anxiety disorder typically anticipate disaster, and are overly concerned about everyday matters such as health issues, money, death, family problems, friend problems or work difficulties. They often exhibit a variety of physical symptoms, including fatigue, fidgeting, headaches, nausea, numbness in hands and feet, muscle tension, muscle aches, difficulty swallowing, bouts of difficulty breathing, trembling, twitching, irritability, sweating, insomnia, hot flashes, and rashes. |

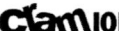

Go to **Cram101.com** for Interactive Practice Exams for this book or virtually any of your books.
And, **NEVER** highlight a book again!

Chapter 12. Antidepressants

Barbiturates	Barbiturates are drugs that act as central nervous system depressants, and, by virtue of this, they produce a wide spectrum of effects, from mild sedation to total anesthesia. They are also effective as anxiolytics, hypnotics and as anticonvulsants. They have addiction potential, both physical and psychological.
Hydroxyzine	Hydroxyzine is a first-generation antihistamine of the piperazine class that is an H_1 receptor antagonist. It was synthesized in the early 1950s. It is used primarily as an antihistamine for the treatment of itches and irritations, an antiemetic for the reduction of nausea, as a weak analgesic by itself and as an opioid potentiator, and as an anxiolytic for the treatment of anxiety.
Meprobamate	Meprobamate is a carbamate derivative which is used as an anxiolytic drug. It was the best-selling minor tranquilizer for a time, but has largely been replaced by the benzodiazepines. Meprobamate was first synthesized by Bernard John Ludwig, PhD, and Frank Milan Berger, MD, at Carter Products in May 1950. Wallace Laboratories, a subsidiary of Carter Products, bought the license and named it Miltown after the village Milltown in New Jersey.
Acamprosate	Acamprosate, also known by the brand name Campral, is a drug used for treating alcohol dependence. Acamprosate is thought to stabilize the chemical balance in the brain that would otherwise be disrupted by alcoholism, possibly by blocking glutamatergic N-methyl-D-aspartate receptors, while gamma-aminobutyric acid (GABA) type A receptors are activated. Reports indicate that Acamprosate only works with a combination of attending support groups and abstinence from alcohol.
Naltrexone	Naltrexone is an opioid receptor antagonist used primarily in the management of alcohol dependence and opioid dependence. It is marketed in generic form as its hydrochloride salt, naltrexone hydrochloride, and marketed under the trade names Revia and Depade. In some countries including the United States, a once-monthly extended-release injectable formulation is marketed under the trade name Vivitrol.
Social anxiety disorder	Social anxiety disorder , is excessive social anxiety (anxiety in social situations) causing considerable distress and impaired ability to function in at least some parts of daily life. The diagnosis can be of a specific disorder (when only some particular situations are feared) or a generalized disorder. Generalized Social anxiety disorder typically involves a persistent, intense, chronic fear of being judged by others and of being embarrassed or humiliated by one's own actions.

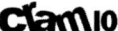

Chapter 12. Antidepressants

Phenotype	A Phenotype is any observable characteristic or trait of an organism: such as its morphology, development, biochemical or physiological properties, or behavior. Phenotypes result from the expression of an organism's genes as well as the influence of environmental factors and possible interactions between the two.
	The genotype of an organism is the inherited instructions it carries within its genetic code.
Pathophysiology	Pathophysiology is the study of the changes of normal mechanical, physical, and biochemical functions, either caused by a disease, or resulting from an abnormal syndrome. More formally, it is the branch of medicine which deals with any disturbances of body functions, caused by disease or prodromal symptoms.
	An alternative definition is 'the study of the biological and physical manifestations of disease as they correlate with the underlying abnormalities and physiological disturbances.'
	The study of pathology and the study of pathophysiology often involves substantial overlap in diseases and processes, but pathology emphasizes direct observations, while pathophysiology emphasizes quantifiable measurements.
Anesthesia	Anesthesia, has traditionally meant the condition of having sensation blocked or temporarily taken away. This allows patients to undergo surgery and other procedures without the distress and pain they would otherwise experience. The word was coined by Oliver Wendell Holmes, Sr.
Ganglion	In anatomy, a ganglion is a biological tissue mass, most commonly a mass of nerve cell bodies. Cells found in a ganglion are called ganglion cells, though this term is also sometimes used to refer specifically to retinal ganglion cells.
	In some dinosaurs, the ganglion in the pelvis was so large relative to its brain that it could almost be said to have two brains.

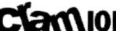

Chapter 12. Antidepressants

Local anesthesia	Local anesthesia is any technique to render part of the body insensitive to pain without affecting consciousness. It allows patients to undergo surgical and dental procedures with reduced pain and distress. In many situations, such as cesarean section, it is safer and therefore superior to general anesthesia.
Spinothalamic tract	The Spinothalamic tract is a sensory pathway originating in the spinal cord. It transmits information to the thalamus about pain, temperature, itch and crude touch. The pathway decussates at the level of the spinal cord, rather than in the brainstem like the posterior column-medial lemniscus pathway and corticospinal tract.
Capsaicin	Capsaicin $_2$CHCH=CH(CH$_2$)$_4$CONHCH$_2$C$_6$H$_3$-4-(OH)-3-(OCH$_3$)) is the active component of chili peppers, which are plants belonging to the genus Capsicum. It is an irritant for mammals, including humans, and produces a sensation of burning in any tissue with which it comes into contact. Capsaicin and several related compounds are called Capsaicinoids and are produced as a secondary metabolite by chili peppers, probably as deterrents against certain herbivores and fungi.
Neurotrophin	Neurotrophins are a family of proteins that induce the survival, development, and function of neurons. They belong to a class of growth factors, secreted proteins that are capable of signaling particular cells to survive, differentiate, or grow. Growth factors such as neurotrophins that promote the survival of neurons are known as neurotrophic factors.
Hypersensitivity	Hypersensitivity refers to undesirable (damaging, discomfort-producing and sometimes fatal) reactions produced by the normal immune system. Hypersensitivity reactions require a pre-sensitized (immune) state of the host. The four-group classification was expounded by P. H. G. Gell and Robin Coombs in 1963.
Sympathetic nervous system	The Sympathetic nervous system is a branch of the autonomic nervous system along with the enteric nervous system and paraSympathetic nervous system. It is always active at a basal level (called sympathetic tone) and becomes more active during times of stress. Its actions during the stress response comprise the fight-or-flight response.

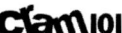

Chapter 12. Antidepressants

Schwann cell	Schwann cells are glia of the peripheral nervous system (PNS). They are involved in many important aspects of peripheral nerve biology; the conduction of nervous impulses along axons, nerve development and regeneration, trophic support for neurons, production of the nerve extracellular matrix and presentation of antigens to T-lymphocytes. Charcot-Marie-Tooth disease (CMT), Guillain-Barré syndrome (GBS), schwannomatosis and chronic inflammatory demyelinating polyneuropathy (CIDP) are all neuropathies involving Schwann cells.
Cytokine	Cytokines are small cell-signaling protein molecules that are secreted by the glial cells of the nervous system and by numerous cells of the immune system and are a category of signaling molecules used extensively in intercellular communication. Cytokines can be classified as proteins, peptides, or glycoproteins; the term 'cytokine' encompasses a large and diverse family of regulators produced throughout the body by cells of diverse embryological origin.
Endorphin	Endorphins are endogenous opioid polypeptide compounds. They are produced by the pituitary gland and the hypothalamus in vertebrates during strenuous exercise, excitement, pain, consumption of spicy food and orgasm, and they resemble the opiates in their abilities to produce analgesia and a feeling of well-being. Endorphins work as 'natural pain relievers.' The term 'Endorphin' implies a pharmacological activity (analogous to the activity of the corticosteroid category of biochemicals) as opposed to a specific chemical formulation.
Phosphorylation	Phosphorylation is the addition of a phosphate (PO_4^{3-}) group to a protein or other organic molecule. Phosphorylation activates or deactivates many protein enzymes. Protein phosphorylation in particular plays a significant role in a wide range of cellular processes.
Histamine	Histamine is a biogenic amine involved in local immune responses as well as regulating physiological function in the gut and acting as a neurotransmitter. Histamine triggers the inflammatory response. As part of an immune response to foreign pathogens, Histamine is produced by basophils and by mast cells found in nearby connective tissues.
Adenosine	Adenosine is a nucleoside composed of a molecule of adenine attached to a ribose sugar molecule (ribofuranose) moiety via a β-N_9-glycosidic bond.

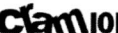

Chapter 12. Antidepressants

	Adenosine plays an important role in biochemical processes, such as energy transfer--as Adenosine triphosphate (ATP) and Adenosine diphosphate (ADP)--as well as in signal transduction as cyclic Adenosine monophosphate, cAMP. It is also an inhibitory neurotransmitter, believed to play a role in promoting sleep and suppressing arousal, with levels increasing with each hour an organism is awake.
	Adenosine is often abbreviated Ado.
Histidine	Histidine Histidine an essential amino acid, has a positively charged imidazole functional group. It is the one of the 22 proteinogenic amino acids. Its codons are CAU and CAC. Histidine was first isolated by German physician Albrecht Kossel in 1896. Histidine is an essential amino acid in humans and other mammals.
Caffeine	Caffeine is a bitter, white crystalline xanthine alkaloid that is a psychoactive stimulant drug. Caffeine was discovered by a German chemist, Friedrich Ferdinand Runge, in 1819. He coined the term kaffein, a chemical compound in coffee, which in English became Caffeine.
	Caffeine is found in varying quantities in the beans, leaves, and fruit of some plants, where it acts as a natural pesticide that paralyzes and kills certain insects feeding on the plants.
Histidine decarboxylase	Histidine decarboxylase is the enzyme that catalyzes the reaction that produces histamine from histidine with the help of vitamin B6 as follows: $$C_6H_9N_3O_2 \rightarrow C_5H_9N_3 + CO_2$$
Ramelteon	Ramelteon, marketed as Rozerem by Takeda Pharmaceuticals North America, is the first in a new class of sleep agents that selectively binds to the MT_1 and MT_2 receptors in the suprachiasmatic nucleus (SCN), versus binding to $GABA_A$ receptors, such as with drugs like zolpidem, eszopiclone, and zaleplon. Ramelteon is approved by the U.S. Food and Drug Administration (FDA) for long-term use.

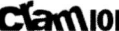

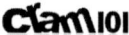

Chapter 12. Antidepressants

	Ramelteon does not show any appreciable binding to $GABA_A$ receptors, which are associated with anxiolytic, myorelaxant, and amnesic effects.
Zolpidem	Zolpidem is a prescription medication used for the short-term treatment of insomnia, as well as some brain disorders. It is a short-acting nonbenzodiazepine hypnotic that potentiates gamma-aminobutyric acid (GABA), an inhibitory neurotransmitter, by binding to gamma-aminobutyric acid ($GABA_A$) receptors at the same location as benzodiazepines. It works quickly (usually within 15 minutes) and has a short half-life (2-3 hours).
Hypnotic	Benzodiazepines are the most well known and most frequently prescribed Hypnotic medication presently. However, their use in recent years is being increasingly replaced by newer nonbenzodiazepine Hypnotic drugs and the hormone melatonin, which in North America is called a 'supplement'. Benzodiazepines are effective in the short term but with long term use beyond 1 - 2 weeks tolerance to their Hypnotic effects develops thus making them ineffective for long term use.
Melatonin	Melatonin , also known chemically as N-acetyl-5-methoxytryptamine, is a naturally occurring compound found in animals, plants, and microbes. In animals, circulating levels of Melatonin vary in a daily cycle, thereby regulating the circadian rhythms of several biological functions. Many biological effects of Melatonin are produced through activation of Melatonin receptors, while others are due to its role as a pervasive and powerful antioxidant, with a particular role in the protection of nuclear and mitochondrial DNA.
	Melatonin in plants has multiple roles, including regulation of the photoperiod, in plant defence responses, and as a scavenger of reactive oxygen species.
Oxidoreductase	In biochemistry, an Oxidoreductase is an enzyme that catalyzes the transfer of electrons from one molecule (the reductant, also called the hydrogen or electron donor) to another (the oxidant, also called the hydrogen or electron acceptor).
Secretion	Secretion is the process of elaborating, releasing, and oozing chemicals, or a secreted chemical substance from a cell or gland. In contrast to excretion, the substance may have a certain function, rather than being a waste product.
	Secretion in bacterial species means the transport or translocation of effector molecules for example proteins, enzymes or toxins (such as cholera toxin in pathogenic bacteria for example Vibrio cholerae) from across the interior (cytoplasm or cytosol) of a bacterial cell to its exterior.

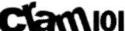

CRAM101

Chapter 12. Antidepressants

Diphenhydramine	Diphenhydramine hydrochloride is a first generation antihistamine mainly used to treat allergies. Like most other first generation antihistamines, the drug also has a powerful hypnotic effect, and for this reason is often used as a non-prescription sleep aid and a mild anxiolytic. The drug also acts as an antiemetic.
Sleep disorders	A sleep disorder (somnipathy) is a medical disorder of the sleep patterns of a person or animal. Some Sleep disorders are serious enough to interfere with normal physical, mental and emotional functioning. A test commonly ordered for some Sleep disorders is the polysomnogram. The most common Sleep disorders include: · Primary insomnia: Chronic difficulty in falling asleep and/or maintaining sleep when no other cause is found for these symptoms. · Bruxism: Involuntarily grinding or clenching of the teeth while sleeping · Delayed sleep phase syndrome (DSPS): inability to awaken and fall asleep at socially acceptable times but no problem with sleep maintenance, a disorder of circadian rhythms. Other such disorders are advanced sleep phase syndrome (ASPS) and Non-24-hour sleep-wake syndrome (Non-24), both much less common than DSPS. · Hypopnea syndrome: Abnormally shallow breathing or slow respiratory rate while sleeping · Narcolepsy: Excessive daytime sleepiness (EDS) often culminating in falling asleep spontaneously but unwillingly at inappropriate times. · Cataplexy, a sudden weakness in the motor muscles that can result in collapse to the floor. · Night terror, Pavor nocturnus, sleep terror disorder: abrupt awakening from sleep with behavior consistent with terror · Parasomnias: Disruptive sleep-related events involving inappropriate actions during sleep stages - sleep walking and night-terrors are examples.

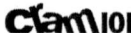

Chapter 12. Antidepressants

· Periodic limb movement disorder (PLMD): Sudden involuntary movement of arms and/or legs during sleep, for example kicking the legs.

Armodafinil	Armodafinil is a stimulant-like drug produced by the pharmaceutical company Cephalon Inc., which was approved by the FDA on June 15, 2007. Armodafinil is an enantiopure drug consisting of just the active (−)-(R)-enantiomer of the racemic drug modafinil (Provigil).
Cataplexy	Cataplexy is a sudden and transient episode of loss of muscle tone, often triggered by emotions. It is a rare disease (prevalence of fewer than 5 per 10,000 in the community), but affects roughly 70% of people who have narcolepsy. Cataplexy can also be present as a side effect of SSRI Discontinuation Syndrome.
Sodium	Sodium is a metallic element with a symbol Na and atomic number 11. It is a soft, silvery-white, highly reactive metal and is a member of the alkali metals within 'group 1' (formerly known as 'group IA'). It has only one stable isotope, ^{23}Na.
Attention deficit hyperactivity disorder	Attention deficit hyperactivity disorder is a developmental disorder. It is primarily characterized by 'the co-existence of attentional problems and hyperactivity, with each behavior occurring infrequently alone' and symptoms starting before seven years of age. Attention deficit hyperactivity disorder is the most commonly studied and diagnosed psychiatric disorder in children, affecting about 3 to 5 percent of children globally and diagnosed in about 2 to 16 percent of school aged children.
Iloperidone	Iloperidone is an atypical antipsychotic for the treatment of schizophrenia. It was approved by the U.S. Food and Drug Administration (FDA) for use in the United States on May 6, 2009.
Alcohol	In chemistry, an Alcohol is any organic compound in which a hydroxyl group (-OH) is bound to a carbon atom of an alkyl or substituted alkyl group. An important group of Alcohols is formed by the simple acyclic Alcohols, the general formula for which is $C_nH_{2n+1}OH$. Of those, ethanol (C_2H_5OH) is the type of Alcohol found in Alcoholic beverages, and in common speech the word Alcohol means, specifically, ethanol. Other Alcohols are usually described with a clarifying adjective, as in isopropyl Alcohol or wood Alcohol.

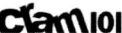

CLam101

Chapter 12. Antidepressants

Guanfacine	Guanfacine has the cardiovascular effect of lowering blood pressure. It does not affect heart rate but significantly reduces hypertension not just in short-term, but also as shown in long-term studies with normalization of blood pressure of 54% treated over a year and 66% over two years. It is also effective in treating the symptoms of attention-deficit hyperactivity disorder (ADHD) as an alternative to stimulants.
Tianeptine	Tianeptine is a selective serotonin reuptake enhancer (SSRE) drug used for treating Major depressive episodes (mild, moderate, or severe). Unlike conventional tricyclic antidepressants, Tianeptine enhances the reuptake of serotonin instead of inhibiting it, opposite to the action of SSRIs. Moreover, it enhances the extracellular concentration of dopamine in the nucleus accumbens.
Stimulants	Stimulants, also sometimes called psychoStimulants, are psychoactive drugs which induce temporary improvements in either mental or physical function or both. Examples of these kinds of effects may include enhanced alertness, wakefulness, and locomotion, among others. Due to their effects typically having an 'up' quality to them, Stimulants are also occasionally referred to as 'uppers'.
Dementia	Dementia is a serious cognitive disorder. It may be static, the result of a unique global brain injury or progressive, resulting in long-term decline in cognitive function due to damage or disease in the body beyond what might be expected from normal aging. Although Dementia is far more common in the geriatric population, it may occur in any stage of adulthood.
Neurofibrillary tangle	Neurofibrillary Tangles are aggregates of hyperphosphorylated tau protein that are most commonly known as a primary marker of Alzheimer's Disease. Their presence is also found in numerous other diseases known as Tauopathies. Little is known about their exact relationship to the different pathologies.
Astrocyte	Astrocytes are characteristic star-shaped glial cells in the brain and spinal cord. They perform many functions, including biochemical support of endothelial cells which form the blood-brain barrier, provision of nutrients to the nervous tissue, maintenance of extracellular ion balance, and a principal role in the repair and scarring process of the brain and spinal cord following traumatic injuries.

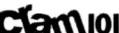

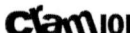

Chapter 12. Antidepressants

	Research since the mid-1990s has shown that Astrocytes propagate intercellular Ca^{2+} waves over long distances in response to stimulation, and, similar to neurons, release transmitters (called gliotransmitters) in a Ca^{2+}-dependent manner.
Oligomer	In chemistry, an oligomer is a molecule that consists of a few monomer units, in contrast to a polymer that, at least in principle, consists of an unlimited number of monomers. Dimers, trimers and tetramers are oligomers. Many oils are oligomeric, such as liquid paraffin.
Presenilin	Presenilins are a family of related multi-pass transmembrane proteins that function as a part of the gamma-secretase protease complex. Vertebrates have two Presenilin genes, called PSEN1 (located on chromosome 14 in humans) that encodes Presenilin 1 (PS-1) and PSEN2 (on chromosome 1 in humans) that codes for Presenilin 2 (PS-2). Both genes show conservation between species, with little difference between rat and human Presenilins.
Transferase	In biochemistry, a Transferase is an enzyme that catalyzes the transfer of a functional group (e.g. a methyl or phosphate group) from one molecule (called the donor) to another (called the acceptor). For example, an enzyme that catalyzed this reaction would be a Transferase: A-X + B → A + B-X In this example, A would be the donor, and B would be the acceptor. The donor is often a coenzyme.
Acetylcholinesterase	Acetylcholinesterase is an enzyme that degrades (through its hydrolytic activity) the neurotransmitter acetylcholine, producing choline and an acetate group. It is mainly found at neuromuscular junctions and cholinergic nervous system, where its activity serves to terminate synaptic transmission. Acetylcholinesterase has a very high catalytic activity -- each molecule of Acetylcholinesterase degrades about 25000 molecules of acetylcholine per second.
Insulin	insulin is a hormone that has extensive effects on metabolism and other body functions, such as vascular compliance. insulin causes cells in the liver, muscle, and fat tissue to take up glucose from the blood, storing it as glycogen in the liver and muscle, and stopping use of fat as an energy source. When insulin is absent (or low), glucose is not taken up by body cells, and the body begins to use fat as an energy source, for example, by transfer of lipids from adipose tissue to the liver for mobilization as an energy source.

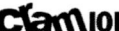

Chapter 12. Antidepressants

Nicotinic	Nicotinic acetylcholine receptors, are cholinergic receptors that form ligand-gated ion channels in the plasma membranes of certain neurons. Being ionotropic receptors, nAChRs are directly linked to an ion channel and do not make use of a second messenger as metabotropic receptors do.
	Like the other type of acetylcholine receptors - muscarinic acetylcholine receptors (mAChRs) - the nAChR is triggered by the binding of the neurotransmitter acetylcholine (ACh).
Cholinesterase	In biochemistry, Cholinesterase is a family of enzymes that catalyze the hydrolysis of the neurotransmitter acetylcholine into choline and acetic acid, a reaction necessary to allow a cholinergic neuron to return to its resting state after activation.
	There are two types:
	· AcetylCholinesterase (AChE), also known as RBC Cholinesterase, erythrocyte Cholinesterase, or (most formally) acetylcholine acetylhydrolase, found primarily in the blood and neural synapses
	· PseudoCholinesterase (BChE or BuChE), also known as plasma Cholinesterase, butyrylCholinesterase, or (most formally) acylcholine acylhydrolase, found primarily in the liver. The difference between the two types of Cholinesterase has to do with their respective preferences for substrates: the former hydrolyses acetylcholine more quickly; the latter hydrolyses butyrylcholine more quickly.
	In 1968, Walo Leuzinger et al.
Cholinesterase inhibitor	An acetylCholinesterase inhibitor or anti-cholinesterase is a chemical that inhibits the cholinesterase enzyme from breaking down acetylcholine, increasing both the level and duration of action of the neurotransmitter acetylcholine.
	AcetylCholinesterase inhibitors:
	· Occur naturally as venoms and poisons

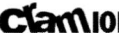

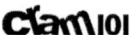

Chapter 12. Antidepressants

· Are used as weapons in the form of nerve agents

· Are used medicinally:

· To treat myasthenia gravis. In myasthenia gravis, they are used to increase neuromuscular transmission.

· To treat Alzheimer's disease

· To treat Lewy Body Dementia

· As an antidote to anticholinergic poisoning

Compounds which function as reversible competitive or noncompetitive inhibitors of cholinesterase are those most likely to have therapeutic uses. These include:

· Organophosphates

· Metrifonate (irreversible)

· Carbamates

· Physostigmine

· Neostigmine

· Pyridostigmine

· Ambenonium

· Demarcarium

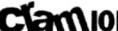

· Rivastigmine

· Phenanthrene derivatives

· Galantamine

· Piperidines

· Donepezil, also known as E2020

· Tacrine, also known as tetrahydroaminoacridine (THA')

· Edrophonium

· Huperzine A

· Ladostigil

Compounds which function as quasi-irreversible inhibitors of cholinesterase are those most likely to have use as chemical weapons or pesticides. These include:

· Huperzine A

· Galantamine

· Onchidal

Some major effects of Cholinesterase inhibitors:

(none)

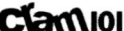

Chapter 12. Antidepressants

	· Actions on the autonomic nervous system, that is parasympathetic nervous system will cause bradycardia, hypotension, hypersecretion, bronchoconstriction, GI tract hypermotility, and decrease intraocular pressure. · SLUDGE syndrome. · Actions on the neuromuscular junction will result in prolonged muscle contraction. When used in the central nervous system to alleviate neurological symptoms, such as rivastigmine in Alzheimer's disease, all Cholinesterase inhibitors require doses to be increased gradually over several weeks, and this is usually referred to as the titration phase.
Donepezil	Donepezil marketed under the trade name Aricept by its developer Eisai and partner Pfizer, is a centrally acting reversible acetylcholinesterase inhibitor. Its main therapeutic use is in the treatment of Alzheimer's disease where it is used to increase cortical acetylcholine. Its binding to the acetylcholinesterase can be seen at Proteopedia 1eve.
Tacrine	Tacrine is a parasympathomimetic and a centrally acting cholinesterase inhibitor (anticholinesterase). It was the first centrally-acting cholinesterase inhibitor approved for the treatment of Alzheimer's disease, and was marketed under the trade name Cognex. Tacrine was first synthesised by Adrien Albert at the University of Sydney.
Rivastigmine	Rivastigmine is a parasympathomimetic or cholinergic agent for the treatment of mild to moderate dementia of the Alzheimer's type and dementia due to Parkinson's disease. The drug can be administered orally or via a transdermal patch; the latter form reduces the prevalence of side effects, which typicaly include nausea and vomiting. The drug is eliminated through the urine, and appears to have relatively few drug-drug interactions.
Galantamine	Galantamine is a chemical used for the treatment of mild to moderate Alzheimer's disease and various memory impairments. It is an alkaloid that is obtained synthetically or from the bulbs and flowers of the Caucasian snowdrop (Voronov's snowdrop), Galanthus woronowii (Amaryllidaceae) and related genera like Narcissus (daffodil), Leucojum (snowflake) and Lycoris including Lycoris radiata (Red Spider Lily). The active ingredient was isolated by prof.
Mechanism of action	In pharmacology, the term Mechanism of action refers to the specific biochemical interaction through which a drug substance produces its pharmacological effect. A Mechanism of action usually includes mention of the specific molecular targets to which the drug binds, such as an enzyme or receptor.

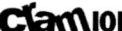

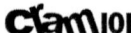

Chapter 12. Antidepressants

	For example, the Mechanism of action of aspirin involves irreversible inhibition of the enzyme cyclooxygenase, which suppresses the production of prostaglandins and thromboxanes, thereby reducing pain and inflammation.
Vitamin E	vitamin E is a generic term for tocopherols and tocotrienols. vitamin E is a family of α-, β-, γ-, and δ-tocopherols and corresponding four tocotrienols. vitamin E is a fat-soluble antioxidant that stops the production of reactive oxygen species formed when fat undergoes oxidation.
Rosiglitazone	Rosiglitazone is an anti-diabetic drug in the thiazolidinedione class of drugs. It is marketed by the pharmaceutical company GlaxoSmithKline as a stand-alone drug (Avandia) and in combination with metformin (Avandamet) or with glimepiride (Avandaryl). Annual sales peaked at approx $2.5bn in 2006. The drug's patent expires in 2012.
Statins	The statins are a class of drugs that lower cholesterol levels in people. They lower cholesterol by inhibiting the enzyme HMG-CoA reductase, which is the rate-limiting enzyme of the mevalonate pathway of cholesterol synthesis. Inhibition of this enzyme in the liver results in decreased cholesterol synthesis as well as increased synthesis of LDL receptors, resulting in an increased clearance of low-density lipoprotein (LDL) from the bloodstream.
Vaccine	A vaccine is a biological preparation that improves immunity to a particular disease. A vaccine typically contains an agent that resembles a disease-causing microorganism, and is often made from weakened or killed forms of the microbe. The agent stimulates the body's immune system to recognize the agent as foreign, destroy it, and 'remember' it, so that the immune system can more easily recognize and destroy any of these microorganisms that it later encounters.
Fluphenazine	Fluphenazine is a typical antipsychotic drug used for the treatment of psychoses such as schizophrenia and acute manic phases of bipolar disorder. It belongs to the piperazine class of phenothiazines and is extremely potent; more potent than haloperidol and around fifty to seventy times the potency of chlorpromazine. Its main use is as a long acting injection given once every two or three weeks to people with schizophrenia who have a poor compliance with medication and suffer frequent relapses of illness.

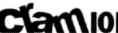

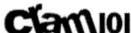

Chapter 12. Antidepressants

Valproate semisodium	Valproate semisodium or divalproex sodium (USAN) consists of a compound of sodium valproate and valproic acid in a 1:1 molar relationship in an enteric coated form. It is used in the UK, Canada, and U.S. for the treatment of the manic episodes of bipolar disorder. In rare cases, it is also used as a treatment for major depressive disorder, and increasingly taken long-term for prevention of both manic and depressive phases of bipolar disorder, especially the rapid-cycling variant.
Addiction	The term 'addiction' is used in many contexts to describe an obsession, compulsion, or excessive psychological dependence, such as: drug addiction problem gambling, crime, money, work addiction, compulsive overeating, Oniomania (compulsive shopping), computer addiction, video game addiction, pornography addiction, television addiction, etc.
	In medical terminology, an addiction is a chronic neurobiologic disorder that has genetic, psychosocial, and environmental dimensions and is characterized by one of the following: the continued use of a substance despite its detrimental effects, impaired control over the use of a drug (compulsive behavior), and preoccupation with a drug's use for non-therapeutic purposes (i.e. craving the drug). addiction is often accompanied by the presence of deviant behaviors (for instance stealing money and forging prescriptions) that are used to obtain a drug.
Cross-tolerance	Cross-tolerance refers to a pharmacological phenomenon, in which a patient being treated with a drug exhibits a physiological resistance to that medication as a result of tolerance to a pharmacologically similar drug. In other words, there is a decrease in response to one drug due to exposure to another drug. It is observed in treatment with antivirals, antibiotics, analgesics and many other medications.
Dopamine antagonist	A Dopamine antagonist is a drug which blocks dopamine receptors by receptor antagonism. There are five known types of dopamine receptors in the human body; they are found in the brain, peripheral nervous system, blood vessels, and the kidney.
	· Used as atypical antipsychotics (coupled with serotonin antagonist effects): clozapine, risperidone, olanzapine, quetiapine, and ziprasidone
	· Used as antiemetics: metoclopramide, droperidol, domperidone
	· Used as tricyclic antidepressants: amoxapine

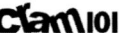

· parkinsonism - due to effects on the nigrostriatal pathway

· hyperprolactinaemia - due to effects on the tuberoinfundibular pathway

· tardive dyskinesia (long term use)
Other examples include:

· acepromazine

· amisulpride

· amoxapine

· azaperone

· benperidol

· bromopride

· butaclamol

· chlorpromazine

· chlorprothixene

· clopenthixol

· domperidone

· droperidol

· eticlopride

· flupenthixol

· fluphenazine

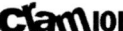

· fluspirilene

· haloperidol

· loxapine

· mesoridazine

· levomepromazine

· metoclopramide

· nafadotride

· nemonapride

· penfluridol

· perazine

· perphenazine

· pimozide

· prochlorperazine

· promazine

· raclopride

· remoxipride

· risperidone

· spiperone

· spiroxatrine

· stepholidine

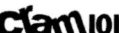

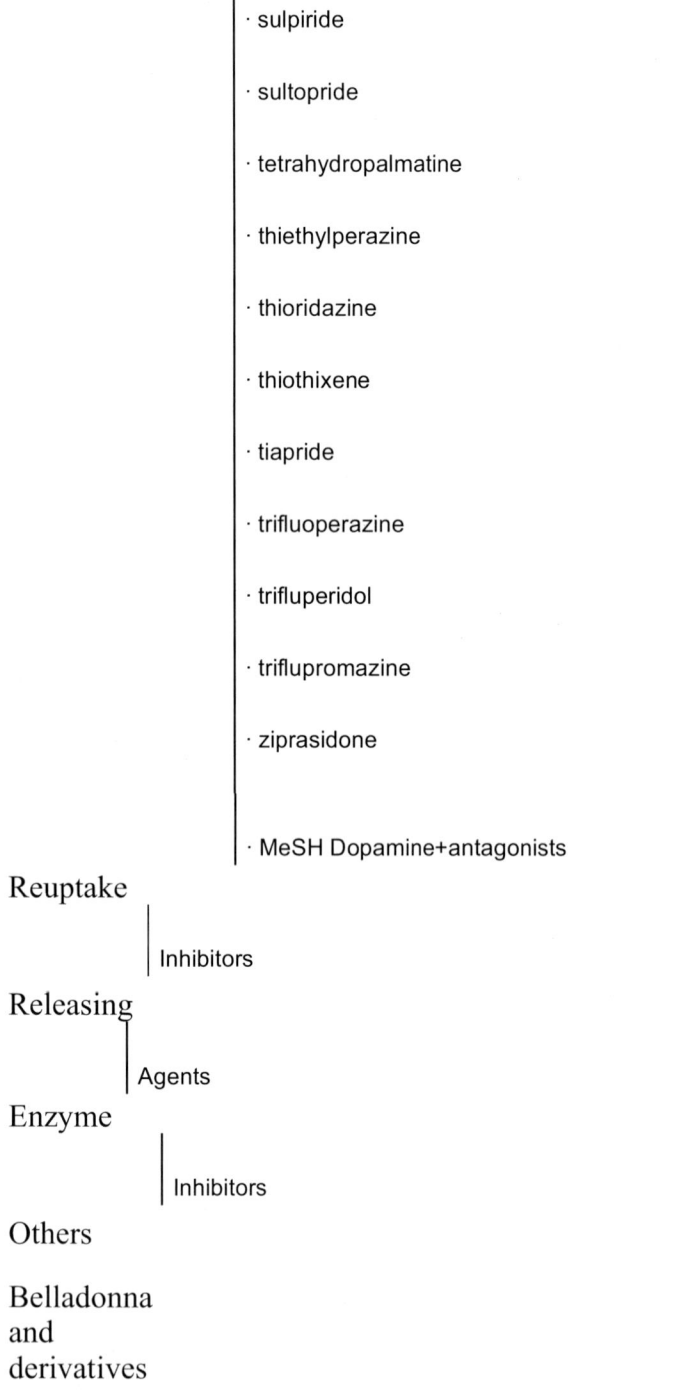

· sulpiride

· sultopride

· tetrahydropalmatine

· thiethylperazine

· thioridazine

· thiothixene

· tiapride

· trifluoperazine

· trifluperidol

· triflupromazine

· ziprasidone

· MeSH Dopamine+antagonists

Reuptake

Inhibitors

Releasing

Agents

Enzyme

Inhibitors

Others

Belladonna
and
derivatives

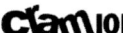

.

(antimuscarinics)

Propulsives

Hallucinogens	The general group of pharmacological agents commonly known as Hallucinogens can be divided into three broad categories: psychedelics, dissociatives, and deliriants. These classes of psychoactive drugs have in common that they can cause subjective changes in perception, thought, emotion and consciousness. Unlike other psychoactive drugs, such as stimulants and opioids, the Hallucinogens do not merely amplify familiar states of mind, but rather induce experiences that are qualitatively different from those of ordinary consciousness.
Varenicline	Varenicline is a prescription medication used to treat smoking addiction. Varenicline is a nicotinic receptor partial agonist. In this respect, it is similar to cytisine and different from the nicotinic antagonist, bupropion, and nicotine replacement therapies (NRTs) like nicotine patches (commonly, 'the patch') and nicotine gum.
Rimonabant	Rimonabant is an anorectic anti-obesity drug. It is an inverse agonist for the cannabinoid receptor CB1. Its main avenue of effect is reduction in appetite. Rimonabant was the first selective CB1 receptor blocker to be approved for use anywhere in the world.
Nalmefene	Nalmefene (Revex) is an opioid receptor antagonist used primarily in the management of alcohol dependence, and also has been investigated for the treatment of other addictions such as pathological gambling and addiction to shopping. Nalmefene is an opiate derivative similar in both structure and activity to the opiate antagonist naltrexone. Advantages of Nalmefene relative to naltrexone include longer half life, greater oral bioavailability and no observed dose-dependent liver toxicity.
Theophylline	Theophylline, also known as dimethylxanthine, is a methylxanthine drug used in therapy for respiratory diseases such as COPD or asthma under a variety of brand names. Due to its numerous side-effects, these drugs are now rarely administered for clinical use. As a member of the xanthine family, it bears structural and pharmacological similarity to caffeine.
Codeine	Codeine (INN) or methylmorphine is an opiate used for its analgesic, antitussive, and antidiarrheal properties.

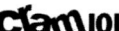

Chapter 12. Antidepressants

	Codeine is an alkaloid found in opium and other poppy saps like Papaver bracteatum, the Iranian poppy, in concentrations ranging from 0.3 to 3.0 percent. While Codeine can be extracted from opium, most Codeine is synthesized from morphine through the process of O-methylation.
Disulfiram	Disulfiram is a drug used to support the treatment of chronic alcoholism by producing an acute sensitivity to alcohol. Trade names for Disulfiram in different countries are Antabuse and Antabus manufactured by Odyssey Pharmaceuticals. Disulfiram is also being studied as a treatment for cocaine dependence, as it prevents the breakdown of dopamine (a neurotransmitter whose release is stimulated by cocaine); the excess dopamine results in increased anxiety, higher blood pressure, restlessness and other unpleasant symptoms.
Morphine	Morphine is a potent opiate analgesic psychoactive drug and is considered to be the prototypical opioid. In clinical medicine, Morphine is regarded as the gold standard, or benchmark, of analgesics used to relieve severe or agonizing pain and suffering. Like other opioids, e.g. oxycodone , hydromorphone , and diacetylMorphine, Morphine acts directly on the central nervous system (CNS) to relieve pain.
Ondansetron	Ondansetron is a serotonin 5-HT$_3$ receptor antagonist used mainly as an antiemetic to treat nausea and vomiting, often following chemotherapy. Its effects are thought to be on both peripheral and central nerves. Ondansetron reduces the activity of the vagus nerve, which deactivates the vomiting center in the medulla oblongata, and also blocks serotonin receptors in the chemoreceptor trigger zone.
Sodium channel	Sodium channels are integral membrane proteins that form ion channels, conducting sodium ions (Na$^+$) through a cell's plasma membrane. They are classified according to the trigger that opens the channel for such ions, i.e. either a voltage-change (voltage-gated Sodium channels) or binding of a substance (a ligand) to the channel (ligand-gated Sodium channels). In excitable cells such as neurons, myocytes, and certain types of glia, Sodium channels are responsible for the rising phase of action potentials.
Cold turkey	'Cold turkey' is an expression describing the actions of a person who gives up a habit or addiction all at once. That is, rather than gradually easing the process through reduction or by using replacement medication. Its supposed advantage is that by not actively using supplemental methods, the person avoids thinking about the habit and its temptation, and avoids further feeding the chemical addiction.

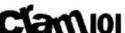

Chapter 12. Antidepressants

Buprenorphine	Buprenorphine is a semi-synthetic opiate with partial agonist actions at the mu opioid receptor and antagonist actions at other opioid receptors. Buprenorphine hydrochloride was first marketed in the 1980s by Reckitt ' Colman (now Reckitt Benckiser) as an analgesic, available generally as Temgesic 0.2 mg sublingual tablets, and as Buprenex in a 0.3 mg/ml injectable formulation. In October 2002, the Food and Drug Administration (FDA) of the United States of America additionally approved Suboxone and Subutex, Buprenorphine's high-dose sublingual pill preparations for opioid addiction, and as such the drug is now also used for this purpose.
Methadone	Methadone is a synthetic opioid, used medically as an analgesic, antitussive and a maintenance anti-addictive for use in patients on opioids. It was developed in Germany in 1937. Although chemically unlike morphine or heroin, Methadone also acts on the opioid receptors and thus produces many of the same effects. Methadone is also used in managing chronic pain owing to its long duration of action and very low cost.
Naloxone	Naloxone is a drug used to counter the effects of opioid overdose, for example heroin or morphine overdose. Naloxone is specifically used to counteract life-threatening depression of the central nervous system and respiratory system. Naloxone is also experimentally used in the treatment for CIPA; an extremely rare disorder (1 in 125 million) that renders one unable to feel pain.
Cannabinoid	Cannabinoids are a group of terpenophenolic compounds present in Cannabis (Cannabis sativa L) and which occur naturally in the nervous and immune systems of animals. The broader definition of Cannabinoids refers to a group of substances that are structurally related to tetrahydrocannabinol (THC) or that bind to Cannabinoid receptors. The chemical definition encompasses a variety of distinct chemical classes: the classical Cannabinoids structurally related to THC, the nonclassical Cannabinoids, the aminoalkylindoles, the eicosanoids related to the endoCannabinoids, 1,5-diarylpyrazoles, quinolines and arylsulphonamides and additional compounds that do not fall into these standard classes but bind to Cannabinoid receptors.
Cannabinoid receptors	The Cannabinoid receptors are a class of cell membrane receptors under the G-protein coupled receptor superfamily. Cannabinoid receptors are activated by ligands, which are lipid compounds known collectively as cannabinoids. Further distinction of these ligands separates endogenous cannabinoids (endocannabinoids), which are generated naturally inside the body, from exogenous cannabinoids, which are introduced into the body as cannabis or a related synthetic compound.
Haloperidol	Haloperidol is a typical antipsychotic. It is in the butyrophenone class of antipsychotic medications and has pharmacological effects similar to the phenothiazines.

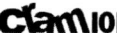

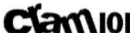
	Haloperidol is an older antipsychotic used in the treatment of schizophrenia and, more acutely, in the treatment of acute psychotic states and delirium.
Designer drug	Designer drug is a term used to describe drugs which are created (or marketed, if they had already existed) to get around existing drug laws, usually by modifying the molecular structures of existing drugs to varying degrees, or less commonly by finding drugs with entirely different chemical structures that produce similar subjective effects to illegal recreational drugs. The term Designer drug also technically applies to the new psychiatric medications, such as the SSRI's and atypical anti-psychotics, as they are designed over many years using testing in animals and neuro-imaging.
Dimethyltryptamine	N,N-Dimethyltryptamine is a naturally occurring psychedelic compound of the tryptamine family. DMT is found not only in several plants, but also in trace amounts in humans and other mammals, where it is originally derived from the essential amino acid tryptophan, and ultimately produced by the enzyme INMT during normal metabolism. The natural function of its widespread presence remains undetermined.
Mescaline	Mescaline or 3,4,5-trimethoxyphenethylamine is a naturally occurring psychedelic alkaloid of the phenethylamine class. It is mainly used as an entheogen, and a tool to supplement various practices for transcendence, including in meditation, psychonautics, art projects, and psychedelic psychotherapy.
	It occurs naturally in the peyote cactus (Lophophora williamsii), the San Pedro cactus (Echinopsis pachanoi) and the Peruvian Torch cactus (Echinopsis peruviana), and in a number of other members of the Cactaceae.
Phentermine	Phentermine, a contraction of 'phenyl-tertiary-butylamine', is an appetite suppressant of the amphetamine and phenethylamine class.
	It is approved as an appetite suppressant to help reduce weight in obese patients when used short-term and combined with exercise, diet, and behavioral modification. It is typically prescribed for individuals who are at increased medical risk because of their weight and works by helping to release certain chemicals in the brain that control appetite.

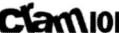

Chapter 12. Antidepressants

Psilocybin	Psilocybin is a hallucinogenic (entheogenic, psychedelic) indole of the tryptamine family. It is produced by hundreds of species of fungi, including those of the genus Psilocybe, such as Psilocybe cubensis and Psilocybe semilanceata, and has also been reportedly isolated from about a dozen other genera. Collectively known as Psilocybin mushrooms, these are commonly called 'boomers,' 'sacred mushrooms,' 'magic mushrooms,' or more simply 'shrooms.' Possession, and in some cases usage, of Psilocybin or psilocin has been outlawed in most countries across the globe.
Psychotomimetic	A drug with Psychotomimetic actions mimics the symptoms of psychosis, including delusions and/or hallucinations. Some drugs of the opioid class have Psychotomimetic effects such as pentazocine and butorphanolX' to describe the effects of the drug marijuana.
Club drugs	Club drugs are a loosely-defined category of recreational drugs which are associated with discothèques in the 1970s and dance clubs, parties, and raves in the 1980s to the 2000s.
Inhalant	Inhalants are a broad range of drugs in the forms of gases, aerosols including organic solvents (found in cleaning products, fast-drying glues, and nail polish removers), fuels (gasoline (petrol) and kerosene) and propellant gases such as freon and compressed hydrofluorocarbons that are used in aerosol cans such as hairspray, whipped cream and non-stick cooking spray.
Erectile dysfunction	Erectile dysfunction is a sexual dysfunction characterized by the inability to develop or maintain an erection of the penis sufficient for satisfactory sexual performance. An erection occurs as a hydraulic effect due to blood entering and being retained in sponge-like bodies within the penis. The process is most often initiated as a result of sexual arousal, when signals are transmitted from the brain to nerves in the pelvis.
Levitra	Vardenafil (INN) is a PDE5 inhibitor used for treating impotence (erectile dysfunction) that is sold under the trade name Levitra. Vardenafil was co-marketed by Bayer Pharmaceuticals, GSK, and SP under the trade name Levitra. As of 2005, the co-promotion rights of GSK on Levitra have been returned to Bayer in many markets outside the U.S. In Italy, Bayer sells vardenafil as Levitra and GSK sells it as Vivanza, thus, because of European Union trade rules, parallel imports might result in Vivanza sold next to Levitra in the

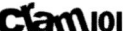

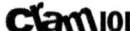

Chapter 12. Antidepressants

	Vardenafil's indications and contra-indications are the same as with other PDE5 inhibitors; it is closely related in function to sildenafil citrate (Viagra) and tadalafil (Cialis).
Sildenafil	Sildenafil citrate, sold as Viagra, Revatio and under various other trade names, is a drug used to treat erectile dysfunction and pulmonary arterial hypertension (PAH). It was developed and is being marketed by the pharmaceutical company Pfizer. It acts by inhibiting cGMP specific phosphodiesterase type 5, an enzyme that regulates blood flow in the penis.
Vardenafil	Vardenafil is a PDE5 inhibitor used for treating impotence (erectile dysfunction) that is sold under the trade name Levitra (Bayer AG, GSK, and SP).
	Vardenafil was co-marketed by Bayer Pharmaceuticals, GSK, and SP under the trade name Levitra. As of 2005, the co-promotion rights of GSK on Levitra have been returned to Bayer in many markets outside the U.S. In Italy, Bayer sells Vardenafil as Levitra and GSK sells it as Vivanza, thus, because of European Union trade rules, parallel imports might result in Vivanza sold next to Levitra in the
	Vardenafil's indications and contra-indications are the same as with other PDE5 inhibitors; it is closely related in function to sildenafil citrate (Viagra) and tadalafil (Cialis).
Erection	Penile erection is a physiological phenomenon where the penis becomes enlarged and firm. Penile erection is the result of a complex interaction of psychological, neural, vascular and endocrine factors, and is usually, though not exclusively, associated with sexual arousal. In some males, erection can occur spontaneously at any time of day, and is known as nocturnal penile tumescence when occurring during rapid eye movement sleep.
Prostaglandin	A prostaglandin is any member of a group of lipid compounds that are derived enzymatically from fatty acids and have important functions in the animal body. Every prostaglandin contains 20 carbon atoms, including a 5-carbon ring. They are mediators and have a variety of strong physiological effects, such as regulating the contraction and relaxation of smooth muscle tissue.
Bremelanotide	Bremelanotide (formerly PT-141) is a compound under drug development by Palatin Technologies as a treatment for hemorrhagic shock and reperfusion injury. It functions by activating the melanocortin receptors MC1R and MC4R, to modulate inflammation and limiting ischemia. It was originally developed for use in treating sexual dysfunction but this application was discontinued in 2008, after concerns were raised over adverse side effects of increased blood pressure.

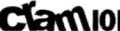

Chapter 12. Antidepressants

Testosterone	Testosterone is a steroid hormone from the androgen group. In mammals, Testosterone is primarily secreted in the testes of males and the ovaries of females, although small amounts are also secreted by the adrenal glands. It is the principal male sex hormone and an anabolic steroid.
Orlistat	Orlistat, also known as tetrahydrolipstatin, is a drug designed to treat obesity. Its primary function is preventing the absorption of fats from the human diet, thereby reducing caloric intake. It is intended for use in conjunction with a physician-supervised reduced-calorie diet.
Metformin	Metformin (INN; trade names Glucophage, Glucophage XR, Riomet, Fortamet, Glumetza, Obimet, Dianben, Diabex, Diaformin, and others) is an oral anti-diabetic drug from the biguanide class. It is the first-line drug for the treatment of type 2 diabetes, particularly in overweight and obese people and those with normal kidney function, and evidence suggests it may be the best choice for people with heart failure. It is also used in the treatment of polycystic ovary syndrome.

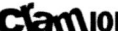

Printed by BoD™in Norderstedt, Germany